T.Myers M4

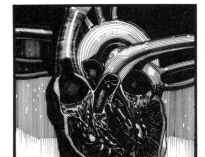

CARDIAC PROBLEMS

Contents

Evaluation

Cardiac Disease

Dysrhythmias

Cardiac Arrest/Cardiac Trauma

Congenital Heart Defects

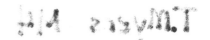

NurseReview

Springhouse Corporation Book Division

Chairman
Eugene W. Jackson

Vice-Chairman
Daniel L. Cheney

President
Warren R. Erhardt

Vice-President, Book Operations
Thomas A. Temple

Vice-President, Production and Purchasing
Bacil Guiley

Program Director
Jean Robinson

Art Director
John Hubbard

Staff

Book Editor
Kathy E. Goldberg

Editors
Katherine W. Carey
Virginia Peck
Patricia Minard Shinehouse

Clinical Editor
Diane Schweisguth, RN, BSN

Drug Information Manager
Larry Neil Gever, RPh, PharmD

Designer
Lynn Foulk Purvis

Illustrators
Julia DeVito
Dan Fione
Robert Jackson

Production Coordinator
Kathleen P. Luczak

Editorial Services Supervisor
David R. Moreau

Copy Editors
Traci A. Deraco
Diane M. Labus
Doris Weinstock

Editorial Assistant
Ellen Johnson

Art Production Manager
Robert Perry

Artists
Mary Braun
Janice Engelke
Donald G. Knauss
Robert Weider

Typography Manager
David C. Kosten

Typography Assistants
Alicia Dempsey
Elizabeth A. DiCicco
Ethel Halle
Diane Paluba
Nancy Wirs

Senior Production Manager
Deborah C. Meiris

Production Manager
Wilbur D. Davidson

Production Assistant
T.A. Landis

Clinical Consultants

Stephen J. Daly, DO
Attending Cardiologist/Director, Cardiac Catheterization Laboratory, Kennedy Memorial Hospitals, University Medical Center, Stratford, N.J.; Assistant Professor of Medicine, University of Medicine and Dentistry-New Jersey School of Osteopathic Medicine, Piscataway

Les Sampson, RN, BSN, CCRN
Nurse Director/Administrator Coordinator, Abington (Pa.) Memorial Hospital

© 1987 by Springhouse Corporation, 1111 Bethlehem Pike, Springhouse, Pa. 19477

NRT1-030590

ISBN 0-87434-103-5

Patient Assessment: History-Taking and Physical Examination

Consider cardiac assessment a cornerstone for good patient care. When done properly, assessment helps identify and evaluate changes in your patient's cardiac function—changes that could disrupt or even threaten his life. A good cardiac assessment yields baseline information that will help guide your intervention and follow-up care.

Even if you don't usually care for patients with cardiac disease, you should know how to identify cardiac problems. In this chapter, we'll review the techniques that'll enhance your cardiac assessment skills.

The nursing history

Begin patient assessment with a thorough nursing history. To take an effective history, rely on your ability to build a rapport with the patient. Ask open-ended questions. Listen carefully to his responses, and closely observe his nonverbal behavior.

Gather the following information when taking a history:

Chief complaint
Ask "What made you seek medical care?" Document the patient's answer in his own words. If he can't identify a single chief complaint, ask more specific questions; for example: "What made you seek medical care at this time?"

Present illness
Ask the patient how long he's had the problem and how it affects his daily routine; when it began; any associated signs and symptoms; location, radiation, intensity, and duration of any pain; and any precipitating, exacerbating, or relieving factors. Let the patient describe his problem in his own words. Avoid leading questions; when possible, use familiar expressions rather than medical terms.

Past medical history
Ask about any history of potentially cardiac-related disorders such as hypertension, diabetes mellitus, hyperlipidemia, congenital heart defects, rheumatic fever, or syncope. Does he use alcohol, tobacco, or caffeine? Does he take any prescription, over-the-counter, or recreational drugs? Find out if the patient's allergic to any drugs, foods, or other agents. If so, have him describe the reaction he's had. Ask a female patient about any pregnancies and find out if she's begun menopause. Does she use oral contraceptives or estrogen? Has she ever had pregnancy-induced hypertension?

Family history
Information about the patient's blood relatives may suggest a specific cardiac problem. Ask him if anyone in his family has ever had high blood pressure, diabetes mellitus, coronary artery disease (CAD), vascular disease, or hyperlipidemia.

Social history
Obtain information about your patient's occupation, educational background, living arrangements, daily activities, and family relationships. Explore any potentially stressful circumstances. Be sure to ask about his exercise habits and diet.

Throughout the history-taking session, note the appropriateness of the patient's responses, his speech clarity, and his mood so that you can identify any later changes.

Virginia Elsenhans, who wrote this chapter, is Adult Medicine Nurse Practitioner at Temple University Medical Practices in Philadelphia. She received her CRNP education from the State University of New York in Syracuse and earned an EdM in community health education from Temple.

Some key questions for assessing cardiac function

To assess your patient's cardiac function, obtain a thorough history. How can you elicit as much information as possible about your patient's signs and symptoms? Avoid leading questions. And when possible, ask questions requiring more than a *yes* or *no* response.

• Do you have any pain? If so, point to the pain site. Describe any chest pain. Do you get a burning or squeezing sensation? What relieves the pain?

• Do you ever feel short of breath? Does a particular body position seem to bring this on? Which one? How long does any shortness of breath last? What relieves it?

• Have you ever awakened suddenly from breathing trouble?

• Do you ever wake up coughing? How often?

• Have you ever coughed up blood?

• Does your heart ever pound or skip a beat? If so, when does this happen?

• Do you ever get dizzy or faint? What seems to bring this on?

• Do your feet or ankles swell? At what time of day? Does anything relieve the swelling?

• Do you urinate more frequently at night?

• Do any activities tire you? Which ones? Have you had to limit your activities or rest more often while doing them?

• Are you less active now than you were 10 years ago? If so, describe the changes.

• Have you ever had severe fatigue not caused by exertion?

• Have you ever been told you have high blood pressure or a heart murmur?

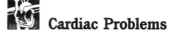

Patient Assessment

Crisis assessment

If the patient's in a cardiac crisis, rethink your priorities. The patient's condition and the clinical situation dictate which assessment steps to take. However, your first goal remains the same—to ensure that his airway, breathing, and circulation are adequate. If any of these seem threatened or compromised, focus on that area and intervene appropriately. Next, check for the following signs and symptoms, which suggest a cardiac problem:

• new onset of chest pain

• chest pain that's unrelieved or increasingly frequent

• chest pain at rest

• change in his level of consciousness

• increased nitroglycerin requirements

• dyspnea at rest, increased orthopnea, or increased exertional dyspnea

• hemoptysis

• unexpected change in cardiac rate or rhythm

• unexpected change in blood pressure

• increased anxiety or restlessness

• diaphoresis or clammy skin.

If you note any of these signs or symptoms, perform an abbreviated assessment using the following steps.

Ask questions phrased so that the patient can answer *yes* or *no*; for example, "Are you having trouble breathing? Do you have chest pain? Are you nauseated, dizzy, or anxious?"

Identify problems. Look for other abnormal changes such as jugular vein distention, increased pallor, cyanosis, or difficulty breathing.

Measure vital signs. Palpate the chest for thrills, lifts, or heaves. Then auscultate heart sounds for rate and rhythm changes and abnormal sounds. At the lung bases, auscultate for crackles.

To remember these steps, think of the mnemonic they form: *AIM (Ask, Identify, and Measure).* Take *AIM,* then act by intervening appropriately. (*Note:* Always assume a patient's signs and symptoms relate to a cardiac problem until proven otherwise.)

Key symptoms

Identifying key symptoms can prove critical to the early recognition of a cardiac problem and its complications. Yet, interpreting these symptoms may not prove easy. A patient with a cardiac problem can have many symptoms—or none at all. And some *apparent* cardiac symptoms can result from other disorders, while symptoms attributed to other body systems may stem from a cardiac problem. Here's what to check for when you suspect a cardiac problem.

Chest pain

Although chest pain's one of the most common symptoms of heart disease, it doesn't always originate in the heart. And sometimes cardiac-related pain appears in areas other than the heart. Pain originating in the heart is transmitted through the thoracic region by the upper five thoracic spinal cord segments, and thus may be referred to areas served by the cervical or lower thoracic segments (such as the neck and arms). Upper thoracic segments innervate skin as well as skeletal muscles, making the true origin of chest pain hard to determine.

Dyspnea

Your patient may describe this symptom as shortness of breath, breathlessness, or difficulty breathing. When dyspnea occurs gradually over weeks and months, it usually suggests a chronic cardiac problem. Look on dyspnea occuring at rest or with slight activity as abnormal. In a patient with a cardiac problem, dyspnea usually results from pulmonary congestion or increased pulmonary venous and capillary pressure. Two types of dyspnea frequently signal cardiac problems. *Orthopnea*—dyspnea that occurs when the patient lies flat—may accompany congestive heart failure. *Paroxysmal nocturnal dyspnea,* which interrupts sleep, commonly disappears when the patient sits upright. It usually results from interstitial pulmonary edema secondary to left ventricular failure. Sudden dyspnea in a patient sitting upright may indicate a myxomatous tumor. In a child, dyspnea relieved by squatting suggests tetralogy of Fallot.

Palpitations

The patient may describe these as heartbeats that seem fast, slow, irregular, forceful, or throbbing. Palpitations can come from smoking, exercise, stress, or excessive intake of beverages containing caffeine. Usually occurring at the cardiac apex, palpitations may also be felt substernally or in the neck. (*Note:* Although palpitations usually develop from cardiac dysrhythmias, not all patients with dysrhythmias have them.)

Syncope

Both syncope (a brief loss of consciousness) and near-syncope (light-headedness or dizziness) develop from inadequate cerebral blood flow. Various cardiac problems can cause syncope, including dysrhythmias, angina, myocardial infarction (MI), aortic stenosis, hypotension, and pacemaker failure. However, syncope and near-syncope sometimes stem from noncardiac disorders.

Edema

When associated with cardiac problems, edema most always arises from increased capillary hydrostatic pressure, which displaces fluid from the capillaries into the tissues. This causes a visibly excessive accumulation of interstitial fluid. Cardiac-related edema may accompany hypertension, left ventricular failure, and increased venous pressure secondary to right heart failure.

Patient Assessment

How various types of chest pain differ

Does your patient complain of chest pain? To accurately assess his cardiac status, find out what type of chest pain he's having. Use the chart below as a guide.

Characteristics	Cause	Location	Aggravating factors	Alleviating factors
CARDIOVASCULAR ORIGIN				
Aching, squeezing, pressure, heaviness, burning; usually subsides within 10 minutes	Angina pectoris	Substernal; may radiate to jaw, neck, arms, and back	Eating, physical effort, smoking, cold weather, stress, anger, hunger, lying down	Rest, nitroglycerin *Note:* Unstable angina appears even at rest
Pressure, burning, aching, tightness; may be accompanied by shortness of breath, diaphoresis, weakness, anxiety, or nausea; sudden onset; lasts ½ to 2 hr	Acute myocardial infarction	Across chest; may radiate to jaw, neck, arms, and back	Exertion, anxiety	Pain is relieved by narcotic analgesics, such as morphine sulfate
Sharp; may be accompanied by friction rub; sudden onset; continuous pain	Pericarditis	Substernal; may radiate to neck, left arm	Deep breathing, supine position	Sitting up, leaning forward, anti-inflammatory agents
Excruciating, tearing; may be accompanied by blood pressure difference between right and left arms; sudden onset	Dissecting aortic aneurysm	Retrosternal, upper abdomen or epigastric; may radiate to back, neck, shoulders	None	Analgesics
PULMONARY ORIGIN				
Sudden, knifelike; may be accompanied by cyanosis, dyspnea, or cough with hemoptysis	Pulmonary embolus	Over lung area	Inspiration	Analgesics
Sudden; severe; may be accompanied by dyspnea, increased pulse, decreased breath sounds, or deviated trachea	Pneumothorax	Lateral thorax	Normal respiration	Analgesics, chest tube
GASTROINTESTINAL ORIGIN				
Dull, pressurelike, squeezing	Esophageal spasm	Substernal, epigastric	Food, cold liquids, exercise	Nitroglycerin, calcium channel blockers
Sharp, severe	Hiatal hernia	Lower chest; upper abdomen	Heavy meal; bending; lying down	Antacids, walking, semi-Fowler position
Burning feeling after eating; may be accompanied by hematemesis or tarry stools; sudden onset; usually subsides within 15 to 20 min	Peptic ulcer	Epigastric	Lack of food or highly acidic foods	Food, antacids
Gripping, sharp; nausea and vomiting may also be present	Cholecystitis	Right epigastric or abdominal areas; may radiate to shoulders	Eating fatty foods, lying down	Rest and analgesics; surgery
MUSCULOSKELETAL ORIGIN				
Sharp; may be tender to the touch; gradual or sudden onset; continuous or intermittent pain	Chest wall syndrome	Anywhere in chest	Movement, palpation	Time, analgesics, heat
OTHER ORIGIN				
Dull or stabbing pain, usually accompanied by hyperventilation or breathlessness; sudden onset; may last less than a minute or for several days	Acute anxiety	Anywhere in chest	Increased respiratory rate; stress or anxiety	Slowing of respiratory rate, stress relief

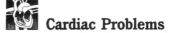

Patient Assessment

What to assess for

Hair: dry and brittle hair may indicate vascular insufficiency or some other heart disease

Ear: diagonal earlobe crease (McCarthy's sign) may indicate coronary artery disease

Head: subtle up-and-down movements in synchronization with heartbeat (Musset's sign) indicate aortic aneurysm or aortic insufficiency

Eyelids: yellow plaque (xanthelasma) may indicate elevated cholesterol

Eye: gray ring at junction of iris and sclera (corneal arcus) indicates hyperlipidemia

Lips and tongue: central cyanosis may indicate oxygen deficiency (hypoxia), cardiac disease, or lung disease

Epigastric area: pulsations in aorta may indicate an abdominal aortic aneurysm

Right upper quadrant: pulsations in liver may indicate tricuspid regurgitation

Elbows: yellow plaque (xanthoma) may indicate elevated cholesterol

Skin color: pallor may mean vasoconstriction; ruddiness may stem from polycythemia; cyanosis suggests oxygen deficiency; Osler's nodes (tender, erythematous lesions on the ends of the fingers or toe pads, palms, and soles) and Janeway spots (nontender hemorrhagic lesions on the palms or soles) may develop from infective endocarditis.

Nailbeds: peripheral cyanosis may indicate peripheral vascular disease or decreased cardiac output

Nails: clubbing may indicate chronic hypoxemia or congenital heart disease; thickness may indicate impaired oxygen delivery to extremities

Skin temperature: cool and dry skin may indicate vascular insufficiency; cool and moist skin may indicate vasoconstriction or anxiety

Lower leg: pretibial edema and pedal edema with pitting may indicate congestive heart failure; without pitting, they may indicate vascular disease

The physical examination

Begin a systematic physical examination of the patient at this point. Using inspection, palpation, percussion, and auscultation, investigate any abnormalities the patient's history or symptoms suggest.

Inspection

First, survey his overall physical condition. Check for acute distress, including airway, breathing, and circulation difficulties; debilitation; and obvious deformities. Then assess the patient's level of consciousness, skin and mucous membranes, jugular veins, carotid artery pulsations, anterior chest, and extremities.

Level of consciousness. Reduced cardiac output can diminish the brain's oxygen supply and alter the patient's consciousness level. Check for such signs and symptoms as restlessness, agitation, and irritability. If inadequate brain oxygenation continues, he may become lethargic, disoriented, confused, and unresponsive.

Skin and mucous membranes. Check for pallor or cyanosis. Pallor occurs when decreased cardiac output or increased sympathetic nervous system activity causes blood vessels to vasoconstrict, shunting blood from the skin to the heart and brain. Sympathetic vasoconstriction also causes peripheral cyanosis—bluish discoloration of the nailbeds, earlobes, and lips. (Central cyanosis, another cyanosis type, causes bluish discoloration of the warm mucous membranes in the nose, mouth, and under the tongue.) However, don't consider cyanosis alone a reliable sign of decreased oxygenation.

Also look for xanthomas (cholesterol-filled nodules on the eyelids and ears), which may accompany hyperlipidemia, and diagonal earlobe creases, commonly seen in infarction patients. In a patient under age 45, these creases suggest CAD.

Jugular veins. Check jugular venous pressure and note any abnormal venous pulsations. Because the jugular veins drain venous blood into the large central veins and eventually into the right atrium, volume or pressure changes in the right atrium can alter volume or pressure in the jugular veins.

Examining jugular venous pulses

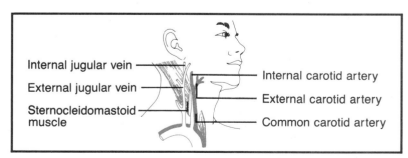

Internal jugular vein
External jugular vein
Sternocleidomastoid muscle
Internal carotid artery
External carotid artery
Common carotid artery

In your cardiac assessment, note the vein and artery distribution in the neck, as shown in this illustration. Observe internal jugular pulsations by shining a flashlight across your patient's neck. This creates reflecting light waves that make his venous pulse visible.

Be sure to distinguish venous pulsations from arterial pulsations and to document your findings carefully.

Patient Assessment

Picturing venous pulsations

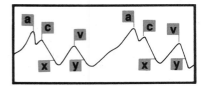

The waveform above shows jugular venous pulsations, as seen on a hemodynamic monitor. These pulsations have *a*, *c*, and *v* waves and *x* and *y* descents. The *a* wave, the first outward pulsation, occurs when a small amount of blood regurgitates into the superior vena cava during right atrial contraction. If atrial contraction doesn't occur, the *a* wave won't appear. A patient with atrial fibrillation, for example, lacks visible *a* waves because his atria don't contract in an organized manner.

Abnormal venous pulsations include accentuated *a* waves, which occur when a closed tricuspid valve prevents atrial blood from draining into the right ventricle. The blood then regurgitates into the venous system, producing a giant *a* wave. Other causes of accentuated *a* waves include dysrhythmias, atrial wall stiffness, right ventricular infarction, right atrial infarction, and right ventricular failure.

Barely visible, the *c* wave is a small outward pulsation that corresponds with ventricular contraction. It occurs on the *a* wave's downstroke.

After atrial contraction and tricuspid valve closure, the right atrium refills with blood. Venous pressure then decreases and the *x* descent appears.

The third outward pulsation, the *v* wave, appears as blood fills the right atrium during atrial diastole.

The *y* descent appears next, as the tricuspid valve opens and blood streams into the right ventricle. Decreased volume and pressure in the right atrium make the blood column in the jugular vein fall, producing the *y* descent.

Diminished *c*-wave amplitude results from decreased right ventricular contractile force secondary to muscle damage. Tricuspid insufficiency can cause an accentuated *cv* wave combination or an absent *x* descent.

To assess jugular venous pulsation, elevate the head of the patient's bed 15° to 45°. Turn the patient's head slightly away from you to relax the sternocleidomastoid muscle so that it doesn't obstruct your view of the veins. With a lamp or flashlight, cast a slight shadow to accentuate the pulsation. Then place a pillow under the patient's head and shoulders. Note any abnormal pulsations.

Next, examine his neck veins to estimate jugular venous pressure. This measurement, which identifies venous distention, indicates right atrial and central venous pressures.

To measure venous pressure indirectly, place the patient at a 45° angle (see illustration below). Observe the internal jugular vein to determine the highest level of visible pulsation. Then locate the angle of Louis, or sternal angle. To do so, palpate the clavicle where it joins the sternum (the suprasternal notch). Place your first two fingers on the notch. Without lifting them from the skin, slide your fingers down the sternum until you feel a bony protuberance—the angle of Louis.

Estimate venous pressure by measuring the vertical distance between the highest level of visible pulsation and the angle of Louis. In most instances, this vertical distance is less than 3 cm. Add 5 cm to this figure to estimate the total distance between the highest level of pulsation and the right atrium. If the total exceeds 10 cm, consider venous pressure elevated and suspect right ventricular failure.

Carotid arteries. Look for hypokinetic (weak) or hyperkinetic (strong and bounding) pulsations. A hypokinetic pulsation may stem from decreased cardiac output. A hyperkinetic pulsation generally occurs in high cardiac output states such as hypoxia, anemia, and anxiety.

Anterior chest. Before inspecting the patient's anterior chest, you'll need to understand the underlying landmarks and cardiac structures. As illustrated on page 8, the sternoclavicular area includes the aorta and its branches (area 1); the aortic area includes the aorta and aortic valve (area 2); the pulmonic area includes the pulmonary artery and pulmonic valve (area 3); the anterior precordium lies over the right ventricle (area 4); the apical area lies over the left ventricle's apex (area 5); the epigastric area reveals

Continued on page 8

Estimating venous pressure

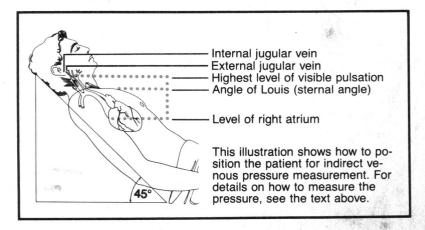

- Internal jugular vein
- External jugular vein
- Highest level of visible pulsation
- Angle of Louis (sternal angle)
- Level of right atrium

45°

This illustration shows how to position the patient for indirect venous pressure measurement. For details on how to measure the pressure, see the text above.

Patient Assessment

How to examine a child

When examining a pediatric patient with a cardiac problem, tailor your assessment to his size and anatomic traits. Consider these points during each examination phase:

Inspection: An infant or a young child breathes with his diaphragm. Assess his breathing pattern by observing his abdomen. Cardiac bulging can mean left ventricular hypertrophy, associated with certain heart defects.

Palpation: In a child under age 4, feel for the point of maximal impulse (PMI) at the third or fourth intercostal space. In older children, you'll find the PMI at the fifth intercostal space.

Percussion: Use very light percussion to identify a child's heart size and location. Heart borders should be triangular.

Auscultation: Expect sinus dysrhythmia, which speeds the heart rate during inspiration and slows it during expiration, in an infant or young child. Ask the child to hold his breath as you auscultate; the sinus dysrhythmia should temporarily disappear.

When listening for heart sounds, you may hear S_3 and systolic murmurs—normal in some children and young adults. Still's murmur, common in children ages 3 to 8, sounds like a vibrating groan or croak. This murmur may arise from occasional vibration of pulmonic leaflets.

Blood pressure reading: When measuring a child's blood pressure, you may have trouble hearing the diastolic sound. In a patient under age 1, you may not hear the systolic sounds either. In this case, use the flush technique to measure blood pressure: elevate the infant's arm or thigh. After the skin blanches, apply the proper size pressure cuff to the infant and inflate it to about 75 mm Hg. Lower the limb and begin deflating the cuff. The pressure reading that appears when the entire limb flushes with color shows the infant's *mean blood pressure.*

Expect a *pulse pressure* of 20 to 50 mm Hg throughout childhood. If it's less than 20 mm Hg, suspect aortic stenosis. If it's more than 50 mm Hg and you've used the proper size pressure cuff, suspect patent ductus arteriosus or aortic regurgitation.

Identifying anterior chest landmarks and structures

When inspecting the patient's anterior chest, check each assessment area (as shown below) for pulsations and abnormal movements.

1-Sternoclavicular area
2-Aortic area
3-Pulmonic area
4-Anterior precordium
5-Apical area
6-Epigastric area
7-Ectopic area

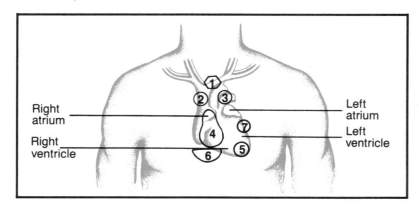

The Physical Examination—*continued*

changes in the liver and abdominal aorta (area 6); and the ectopic area lies over the lateral left ventricular wall (area 7). Inspect each area for pulsations and abnormal movements.

Increased cardiac output or an aortic aneurysm may produce pulsations in the aortic area. Elevated pulmonary artery pressure from left ventricular failure may cause an abnormal pulsation in the pulmonic area. A patient with a thin chest, anemia, increased cardiac output, or anxiety may have slight pulsations to the right and left of the sternum in the anterior precordial area. These abnormalities suggest right ventricular enlargement.

In the apical area, look for a displaced apical impulse or point of maximal impulse (PMI)—the chest region where the left ventricular impulse seems strongest. Displacement sometimes indicates left ventricular enlargement, which may occur secondary to congestive heart failure or systemic hypertension. Also watch for brief outward movement. During diastole, movement suggests a failing left ventricle or mitral insufficiency.

An epigastric pulsation sometimes reflects early signs of congestive heart failure or an aortic aneurysm. However, an ectopic pulsation—even accompanied by chest pain—can be normal.

Next, inspect the patient's chest for deformities and respiratory movement. Thoracic deformities such as kyphosis or scoliosis may restrict lung expansion. Pectus excavatum (funnel chest) and other anterior chest deformities may interfere with closed chest compression.

Also check for respiratory movements that suggest respiratory distress, such as accessory muscle use in the shoulders and neck, intercostal space bulging or retraction, and increased respiratory rate (greater than 20 breaths/minute in adults).

Don't forget that a damaged left ventricle has impaired pumping ability, which in turn increases left ventricle end diastolic blood volume and pressure. This increased pressure affects the left atrium

Patient Assessment

Evaluating edema

These illustrations show how to assess pitting edema. Evaluate your findings on a scale from +1, a barely detectable pit (as shown in the top illustration), to +4, a deep and persistent pit, about 1″ (2.54 cm) deep (see the middle illustration). Some patients accumulate up to 10 lb (4.5 kg) of fluid before edema appears. To assess pitting edema, press firmly for 5 to 10 seconds over a bony surface, such as a subcutaneous part of the tibia, fibula, sacrum, or sternum.

In patients with severe edema, tissue swells so much that fluid can't be displaced, making pitting impossible. The surface tissue feels rock hard as subcutaneous tissue develops fibrosis. This condition may lead to brawny edema (see the bottom illustration).

A lymphatic obstruction can also cause brawny edema. If your patient's extremities show edema, you can help minimize skin sloughing and ulceration by protecting the affected areas from injury.

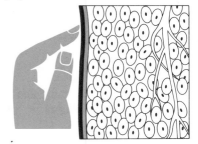

Slight, +1 pitting edema

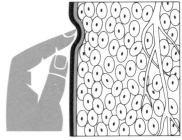

+4 pitting edema

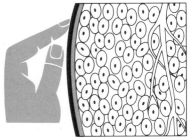

Brawny edema

and pulmonary vein. If pulmonary venous pressure exceeds 22 mm Hg, fluid will shift from the vascular compartments into the pulmonary interstitial space, causing pulmonary edema and eventually respiratory distress. When pulmonary venous pressure increases steadily, severe respiratory distress from intraalveolar edema occurs.

Extremities. Inspect the patient's hands and feet for color changes, clubbing, edema, Osler's nodes, and Janeway spots. Clubbing of the fingers commonly results from hypoxia caused by congenital heart defects or pulmonary disorders. Osler's nodes (tender erythemous lesions on the finger and toe pads, palms, or soles) and Janeway spots (nontender hemorrhagic lesions on the palms and soles) may mean infective endocarditis. *Oslers & Janeway*

Palpation

Use palpation to assess the patient's arterial pulses, extremities, and anterior chest.

Arterial pulses. Palpate all arterial pulses—carotid, brachial, radial, ulnar, femoral, popliteal, dorsalis pedis, and posterior tibial—for presence, rate, rhythm, and quality. Abnormalities suggest vascular problems or provide information about perfusion.

Extremities. Palpate for skin temperature, turgor, and edema. A patient with cool, moist skin could suffer from sympathetic peripheral vasoconstriction caused by decreased cardiac output. If the patient has decreased skin turgor, he may be dehydrated from fluid challenges or potent diuretic therapy. After palpating for edema, rate the amount of edema on a subjective scale from +1 to +4. Edema may occur with right ventricular failure (generalized edema) or left ventricular failure (dependent edema).

Anterior chest. Palpate each chest area for pulsations, thrills, and friction rubs. Use your palm, not your finger pads, to detect prominent pulsations such as heaves or lifts. Forceful beating of an enlarged heart against the sternum or apical area displaces the chest area outward, causing a heave. A palpable murmur produces a thrill. You'll feel a friction rub as a grating or rubbing sensation.

Palpate the apical area to locate the PMI. Normally, the PMI measures less than 2 to 3 cm in diameter, restricted to a single intercostal space. In left ventricular enlargement, however, the PMI's diffuse and displaced to the left midclavicular line below the fifth intercostal space.

Next, palpate the pulmonic area. An abnormal pulsation here may signify increased pulmonary arterial pressure secondary to left ventricular failure. If you palpate a right ventricular lift or heave in the anterior precordial area, suspect right ventricular enlargement.

If you palpate a thrill on the anterior precordium, the patient may suffer from interventricular septal rupture secondary to septal infarction, or tricuspid insufficiency secondary to right ventricular enlargement. A thrill in the apical area suggests mitral insufficiency.

Continued on page 10

Patient Assessment

Auscultatory landmarks

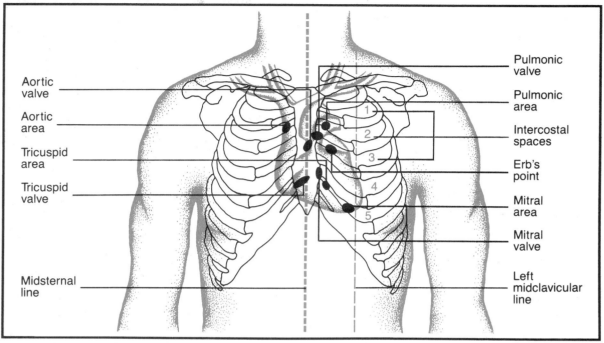

When auscultating for cardiac abnormalities, follow an orderly pattern. First check each heart valve and its related sounds. Then listen, first with the diaphragm and then with the bell, at each valvular area and at Erb's point (as shown in the illustration above).

The Physical Examination—*continued*

A patient who's had an MI may have a palpable outward bulging in the ectopic area during episodes of chest pain. A patient with an aneurysm may have an outward bulging but usually won't have chest pain.

Percussion

Use percussion to outline the heart borders and to determine heart size. Normal cardiac percussion sounds are dull (medium-pitched and muffled, indicating semisolid tissue).

Auscultation

Auscultate for Korotkoff sounds to measure the patient's blood pressure with a sphygmomanometer. Also listen for heart sounds, thought to result from blood accelerating and decelerating in the cardiac chambers, or from blood flow within the heart, great vessels, or both. These sounds arise after heart valve closure.

Auscultate the anterior chest, using a stethoscope with 10″ to 12″ (25.4- to 30.48-cm) tubing. Place the stethoscope's bell lightly on the patient's chest to listen for low-pitched sounds. Use the diaphragm to listen for high-pitched sounds.

Heart valves best transmit sound at the aortic, pulmonic, tricuspid, and mitral area. To hear sounds produced by aortic valve closure, auscultate the second right intercostal space along the right sternal border. You'll hear pulmonic valve sounds at the second left intercostal space along the left sternal border. Listen for tricuspid valve closure at the left sternal border at the fourth or fifth left intercostal space. Expect to hear sounds associated with mitral valve closure at the cardiac apex—the fifth left intercostal space at the midclavicular line. At Erb's point, located at the third left intercostal space along the sternal border, you'll occasionally hear aortic murmurs best.

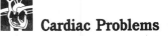
Normal heart sounds

First heart sound (S_1)

S_1 results from the deceleration of blood associated with mitral and tricuspid valve closure. It's usually loudest at the apex (mitral area).

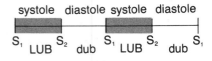

Second heart sound (S_2)

S_2 arises from vibrations produced as the aortic and pulmonic valves close. It's usually heard best at the base of the heart (pulmonic or aortic area).

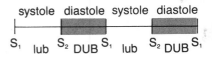

Third heart sound (S_3)

S_3 (ventricular gallop), heard early in diastole, results from vibrations produced during rapid, early ventricular filling into a dilated ventricle. Usually pathologic in the adult, it's commonly heard in children and young adults. Any maneuver that increases venous return (such as exercise or raising the legs) may accentuate the gallop.

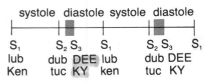

Fourth heart sound (S_4)

S_4 (atrial gallop), which stems from vibrations produced in late diastole, develops after atrial contraction forces blood into a ventricle that resists filling. This sound usually indicates heart disease but sometimes occurs in normal hearts.

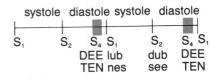

Summation gallop

A summation gallop—the fusing of $S_3 + S_4$—arises from a fast heart rate.

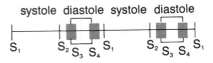

If you detect abnormalities in any valvular area, further evaluate these sounds by listening for sound that's radiated to other chest areas.

The normal heart sounds are S_1 and S_2. S_1 indicates the start of the systolic stage of the cardiac cycle and seems loudest at the apex (mitral area). It comes from blood deceleration as the mitral and tricuspid valves close.

S_2, which marks the beginning of diastole, may sound shorter and louder than S_1. Caused by vibrations produced by aortic and pulmonic valve closure, S_2 seems most audible at the base of the heart (pulmonic or aortic area).

Other heart sounds—S_3, S_4, pericardial friction rubs, splits, opening snaps, ejection clicks, and murmurs—may warn of cardiac abnormalities.

S_3, or ventricular gallop, develops from vibrations that occur during rapid filling into a dilated ventricle. Pathologic in adults, this sound's considered common in children and young adults. Movements that increase venous return may strengthen S_3. Although it signals congestive heart failure, S_3 usually disappears when the rapid-filling disorder resolves. S_3 may also stem from mitral regurgitation, acute left ventricular failure from myocardial ischemia or infarction, and hypertension. You may also notice it with conditions causing volume overload and ventricular dilation, such as mitral, aortic, or tricuspid insufficiency. With right-sided S_3, suspect right heart failure, pulmonary embolism, or pulmonary hypertension.

S_4, or atrial gallop, may result from atrial kick, the vibrations occurring in late diastole after blood flows from the atrium into a ventricle with decreased compliance. This sound frequently indicates systemic hypertension, CAD, cardiomyopathy, or severe aortic stenosis.

Right-sided S_4 may be heard best along the lower left sternal border. Although S_4 usually indicates cardiac disease, you may hear it in a patient with a normal heart.

A summation gallop may develop when a rapid heart rate fuses S_3 and S_4. Arising in middiastole, this sound may best be heard at the cardiac apex.

A pericardial friction rub sounds high-pitched and scratchy, like leather rubbing against leather. This sound occurs when inflammation forces the visceral and parietal surfaces of the pericardium to rub together. Causes include pericarditis, uremia, myocardial infarction, and cardiac surgery. A pericardial friction rub remains unaffected by respiration. It extends through both systole and diastole, coming and going as the pericardial layers make or break contact.

A split develops when one valve closes early or late in relation to the corresponding valve, causing two sounds instead of one.

An opening snap stems from stenotic mitral or tricuspid valve leaflets recoiling abruptly during ventricular diastole.

Movement of a stiff or deformed valve can cause an ejection click.

Patient Assessment

Murmur configurations

To help classify a murmur, identify its configuration (shape). These drawings show the five basic patterns. (Blocks represent heart sounds.)

Crescendo/decrescendo
(diamond-shaped)
Description: Begins softly, peaks sharply, then fades.

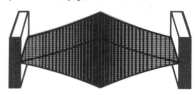

Decrescendo
Description: Starts loudly, then gradually diminishes.

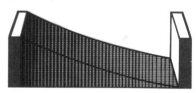

Pansystolic
(holosystolic or plateau-shaped)
Description: Uniform from beginning to end.

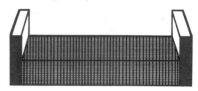

Crescendo
Description: Begins softly, builds gradually.

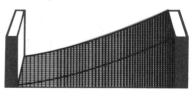

Decrescendo/crescendo
Description: Begins loudly, becomes softer, then builds to original volume.

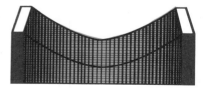

Murmurs

Turbulent blood flow through the heart or the large arteries produces a murmur. A diastolic murmur usually means valvular abnormalities, but a systolic murmur may occur in a healthy heart. Innocent murmurs show up commonly in young children and adults over age 50. They arise from blood flowing forward across normal aortic and pulmonic valves.

Classify murmurs by their timing, configuration, intensity, pitch, quality, location, and radiation.

When *timing* a murmur, determine if it happens during systole or diastole. A murmur occurring between S_1 and S_2 is systolic; between S_2 and the next S_1, diastolic. Also identify whether the murmur comes in early, middle, or late systole or diastole.

To determine a murmur's *configuration*, note the sound's shape, as illustrated at left.

Next, grade the murmur's *intensity* on a scale from I to VI. A grade I murmur's barely audible; a grade II murmur's soft but audible; a grade III murmur's easily audible; a grade IV murmur's loud and associated with a thrill; a grade V murmur, also associated with a thrill, is extremely loud; and a grade VI murmur, the loudest, occurs with a thrill and can be heard without a stethoscope.

A murmur's *pitch* comes from blood flow velocity. To gauge pitch, decide if you can hear the murmur best with the stethoscope's bell (low pitch), with the diaphragm (high pitch), or identically with both (medium pitch).

Describe murmur *quality* as blowing, rasping, harsh, coarse, grating, whistling, or musical. To identify the murmur's *location*, find the area where the sound's loudest. Use anatomical landmarks to define location.

Finally, identify any sound *radiation*. The direction of any radiating sound may provide a clue to the murmur's cause.

Reviewing other body systems

Although you'll focus on the heart when assessing a patient with a suspected cardiac problem, don't overlook potential disorders in other body systems, which can exacerbate a cardiac problem. These findings from other body systems may aid your assessment:
• Neurologic system: decreased level of consciousness, indicating a reduced oxygen supply to the brain
• Respiratory system: crackles, which may signal heart failure; dyspnea, suggesting an increased respiratory rate
• Vascular system: increased or decreased pulse rate, indicating abnormal cardiac output and tissue perfusion; hypertension, possibly indicating CAD
• Renal system: decreased urine output, possibly suggesting abnormal cardiac output or reduced therapeutic effectiveness.

A final note

Once you've completed your baseline assessment, document your findings. You'll refer to them throughout your care. Of course, notify the doctor of any significant changes. But don't stop your assessment there. Continue to assess your patient regularly, using your findings to help determine the cause of any change in his condition.

Diagnostic Tests: Patient Teaching, Preparation, and Nursing Care

Janet Mulligan, a certified critical care nurse in Port Richey, Fla., wrote most of this chapter. She received her MA in adult education, with a specialty in health education, from the University of South Florida in Tampa.

Sharon and John VanRiper contributed the sections on cardiac catheterization, nuclear tests, and magnetic resonance imaging. Sharon, assistant head nurse at the University of Michigan Medical Center in Ann Arbor, received her MS degree from the university. John is a surgical intensive care nurse at the university's Medical Center. He received his BSN degree from Wayne State University in Detroit.

Other Laboratory Tests

The doctor may also order these tests to evaluate your patient's cardiac status:

• *White blood cell count (WBC).* Leukocytosis (increased WBC) may arise just 2 hours after an MI.

• *Erythrocyte Sedimentation Rate (ESR).* A rise in ESR usually follows an MI.

• *Blood glucose.* Hyperglycemia may develop in a patient with coronary artery disease; it may affect up to half of MI patients. (*Note:* For information on cardiac enzyme tests, see Chapter 4.)

Understanding routine diagnostic tests gives you an edge in providing superior care to the patient with a cardiac problem. You won't always take part in the test procedure. But to develop your care plan confidently, you'll want to know why the doctor ordered each test and what test results may mean for your patient. (Of course, always take the patient's clinical status into account when studying test results.)

In this chapter, we'll review diagnostic tests commonly ordered for a patient with a known or suspected cardiac problem—including lab tests and the latest invasive and noninvasive techniques. We'll also explain how to care for the patient before and after the test, and we'll review special nursing considerations. For information about tests that can help diagnose specific cardiac problems, see the chapter describing that problem.

Blood tests

Arterial blood gases (ABGs)
The ABG test measures the efficiency of oxygen and carbon dioxide exchange in the lungs (alveolar ventilation). ABGs also measure the blood's acidity, or pH. An ABG sample is obtained from a percutaneous arterial puncture or drawn from an arterial line.

Interpreting ABG measurements
While reviewing your patient's ABG findings, use the chart below to evaluate his oxygenation, ventilation, and acid-base status.

ABG value	What it measures	Normal values	Significance of abnormal values
pH	Hydrogen ion concentration, blood acidity	7.35 to 7.45	A value greater than 7.45 indicates alkalemia; a value less than 7.35 shows acidemia.
$PaCO_2$	Carbon dioxide tension—the partial pressure exerted by CO_2 dissolved in arterial blood. $PaCO_2$ shows alveolar ventilation.	35 to 45 mm Hg	A value above 45 mm Hg reveals hypoventilation; a value below 35 mm Hg means hyperventilation.
HCO_3^-	Amount of bicarbonate dissolved in the blood, or base excess. Kidneys control HCO_3^- levels; metabolic changes influence this value.	22 to 26 mEq/liter	A value greater than 26 mEq/liter, or a positive base excess value, suggests metabolic alkalosis; a value less than 22 mEq/liter, or a negative base excess value indicates metabolic acidosis.
PaO_2	Oxygen tension—the partial pressure exerted by the small amount of oxygen dissolved in the arterial blood.	80 to 100 mm Hg	A value less than 50 mm Hg means hypoxia. A value between 50 and 80 may indicate hypoxia.
SaO_2	Oxygen saturation, the percentage of hemoglobin carrying oxygen.	95% to 100%	With PaO_2 between 60 and 95 mm Hg, SaO_2 should remain above 85%. Much lower values usually mean a PaO_2 below 50 mm Hg.

Diagnostic Tests

Assessing serum electrolyte and lipid levels

If your patient has a known or suspected cardiac problem, expect the doctor to order any of the tests listed below. Use this chart to review each test's purpose and appropriate nursing considerations.

Serum test and normal values	Test purpose	Nursing considerations
Potassium Normal range: 3.8 to 5.5 mEq/liter	• To detect the origin of cardiac dysrhythmias • To monitor renal function, acid-base balance, and glucose metabolism • To investigate neuromuscular and endocrine disorders	• Check if the patient's receiving diuretics or other drugs that may influence test results. If these medications must be continued, note this on the laboratory slip. • Excessive hemolysis of sample or delay in drawing blood after tourniquet application may elevate serum potassium levels. • Flattened T wave, ST depression, prominent U wave, or PVCs on EKG reveals hypokalemia. • Prolonged PR interval, wide QRS, a tall, tented T wave, or ST depression on EKG suggests hyperkalemia.
Sodium Normal range: 135 to 145 mEq/liter	• To evaluate fluid-electrolyte and acid-base balance and related neuromuscular, renal, and adrenal functions	• Most diuretics decrease serum sodium levels by promoting sodium excretion. • Corticosteroids elevate serum sodium levels by promoting sodium retention. Antihypertensive drugs such as methyldopa, hydralazine, and reserpine may cause sodium and water retention.
Calcium Normal range: 8.9 to 10.1 mg/dl (atomic absorption), or 4.5 to 5.5 mEq/liter. (Expect higher levels in children.)	• To help diagnose cardiac dysrhythmias; neuromuscular, skeletal, and endocrine disorders; blood-clotting deficiencies; and acid-base imbalance	• Prolonged QT interval on EKG suggests hypocalcemia. • Shortened QT interval on EKG suggests hypercalcemia. • Chronic laxative use or excessive transfusions of citrated blood can suppress serum calcium levels. • Excessive vitamin D intake and the use of androgens, dihydrochysterol, calciferol-activated calcium salts, progestins-estrogens, and thiazides can elevate serum calcium levels.
Magnesium Normal range: 1.7 to 2.1 mg/dl (atomic absorption), or 1.5 to 2.5 mEq/liter	• To detect the cause of cardiac dysrhythmias • To evaluate electrolyte status • To assess neuromuscular or renal function	• Tell the patient not to use magnesium salts such as magnesia or Epsom salt for at least 3 days before the test. • Excessive use of antacids or cathartics elevates magnesium levels. • Prolonged I.V. infusions without magnesium may suppress magnesium levels. • Excessive use of diuretics, including thiazides and ethacrynic acid, decreases magnesium levels by increasing urinary magnesium excretion.
Total cholesterol Concentrations vary with age; range: 120 mg/dl to 330 mg/dl	• To measure circulating levels of free cholesterol and cholesterol esters • To assess patient's risk for developing CAD • To evaluate fat metabolism	• Tell the patient to fast overnight and abstain from alcohol for 24 hours before the test.
Triglycerides Normal values vary with age, as follows: 0 to 29 years: 10 to 140 mg/dl 30 to 39 years: 10 to 150 mg/dl 40 to 49 years: 10 to 160 mg/dl 50 to 59 years: 10 to 190 mg/dl	• To screen for hyperlipidemia • To determine patient's risk for developing CAD	• Advise the patient not to eat for 12 hours before the test and to abstain from alcohol for 24 hours before the test.
Lipoprotein-cholesterol fractionation Values vary with age, sex, geographic region, and ethnic group. Check with your hospital's laboratory for normal values	• To assess patient's risk for developing CAD • To isolate and measure major serum lipids: chylomicrons, VLDL, LDL, and HDL	• Advise the patient to abstain from alcohol for 24 hours before the test and to fast and avoid exercise for 12 to 14 hours before the test. • Send the sample to the laboratory immediately to avoid spontaneous redistribution of lipoproteins, which can alter test results.

Diagnostic Tests

What the EKG strip shows

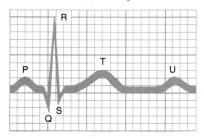

On an EKG strip like the one above, the horizontal axis correlates the length of each particular electrical event with its duration in time. Each small block on the horizontal axis represents 0.04 second. Five small blocks form the base of a large block, which in turn represents 0.20 second.

For more information on EKGs, see Chapter 8.

Electrocardiography (EKG)

This diagnostic method graphically records the heart's electrical activity (electrical potential)—but not its contractions, or mechanical activity. The EKG can identify such disorders as conduction abnormalities, cardiac dysrhythmias, cardiac hypertrophy, pericarditis, electrolyte imbalances, myocardial ischemia, myocardial infarction (MI) site and extent of recovery from an MI. This technique also monitors pacemaker performance and cardiac drug therapy effectiveness. Remember, take into account the patient's clinical status and baseline EKG reading when evaluating EKG results.

Electrodes attached to the patient's chest register the heart's electrical activity. The EKG machine converts this activity into various waveforms and records them on graph paper.

Nursing considerations. Reassure the patient that the EKG won't cause discomfort or electrocution. Because even slight movements, such as shivers or tremors, can reduce an EKG tracing's quality, advise him not to talk or move during the test. Make sure the electrodes make good skin contact.

12-lead EKG

This test helps the doctor evaluate the patient's cardiac disorder by showing the heart's electrical activity from 12 different angles. On a 12-lead EKG tracing, the R wave normally grows taller while the S wave grows shorter when moving from lead V_1 to V_6. The T wave, which normally takes the same direction as the QRS complex in the V leads, if upright, should remain upright. See the chart on page 16 to learn more about the 12-lead EKG.

Exercise EKG

Also known as the stress test, treadmill test, or graded exercise test (GEX), the exercise EKG helps:
• determine how exercise affects chest pain, dysrhythmias, and other cardiovascular signs and symptoms
• determine the prognosis and evaluate the therapy of a patient with coronary artery disease (CAD)
• investigate atypical angina pectoris
• assess peripheral vascular disease and pulmonary function
• gauge a CAD patient's fitness and exercise tolerance
• determine a patient's capacity for work or isometric activities after an anterior MI.

As the patient pedals a stationary bicycle or walks on a treadmill, machines record his EKG waveforms and blood pressure. The test continues until the patient reaches a predetermined target heart rate or has chest pain, fatigue, or other signs and symptoms of exercise intolerance.

Nursing considerations. Tell the patient not to eat or smoke cigarettes for 2 hours before the test. Instruct him to wear comfortable clothing and snug-fitting shoes. Tell him that the test will make him perspire. Encourage him to express any fears he may have. Tell him he can stop the test if he feels chest pain, leg discomfort, or breathlessness.

Holter monitoring

Recording the heart's activity continuously (usually over a 24-hour period), this diagnostic method measures the effects of physical and

Continued on page 16

Diagnostic Tests

Phonocardiography and vectorcardiography

Phonocardiography records heart sounds graphically. Comparing the phonocardiogram with a simultaneous EKG tracing, the doctor can: time events in the cardiac cycle; distinguish murmurs, gallop rhythms, and other abnormal heart sounds; and identify structural valve defects.

Vectorcardiography produces a three-dimensional picture of the heart. The doctor may order this test for a patient with suspected ischemic heart disease or chamber enlargement, MI, or a conduction disturbance.

Electrocardiography—continued

psychological stress on the heart during normal activities. It may also be used for shorter periods; for example, to monitor a patient who has pain or discomfort during a specific activity. The doctor may order Holter monitoring for a patient with intermittent dysrhythmia, dizziness, syncope, chest pain, palpitations, or adverse cardiac reactions to medications. Holter monitoring also helps determine exercise tolerance in post-MI patients; identifies anginal attacks; and helps evaluate the effectiveness of pacemakers and antiarrhythmic and antianginal drugs.

The patient usually wears a tape recorder around his waist. Chest electrodes measure heart current, and the tape records the EKG continuously. After the monitoring period, a computer analyzes the tape and correlates any irregularities with the related activity logged in the diary the patient's instructed to keep.

Nursing considerations. To ensure the best diagnostic results, encourage the patient to update his diary regularly and note any symptoms he has while wearing the monitor. Tell him to perform his normal daily activities. Warn him not to get the monitor wet.

12-lead EKG: A closer look

The EKG's 12 leads each view the heart from a different angle. The chart below lists each lead with corresponding direction of electrical potential and view of the heart. The normal EKG waveforms for each of the 12 leads appear at right.

Views of the heart (left ventricle) reflected on the 12-lead EKG	Leads	Direction of electrical potential	View of heart	Waveform
STANDARD LIMB LEADS (BIPOLAR)				
	I	Between left arm (positive) and right arm (negative)	Lateral wall	I
	II	Between left leg (positive) and right arm (negative)	Inferior wall	II
	III	Between left leg (positive) and left arm (negative)	Inferior wall	III
AUGMENTED LIMB LEADS (UNIPOLAR)				
	aVR	Right arm to heart	Provides no specific view	aVR
	aVL	Left arm to heart	Lateral wall	aVL
	aVF	Left foot to heart	Inferior wall	aVF
PRECORDIAL, OR CHEST, LEADS (UNIPOLAR)				
	V_1	Fourth intercostal space, right sternal border, to heart	Anteroseptal wall	V_1
	V_2	Fourth intercostal space, left sternal border, to heart	Anteroseptal wall	V_2
	V_3	Midway between V_2 and V_4 to heart	Anterior wall	V_3
	V_4	Fifth intercostal space, mid-clavicular line, to heart	Anterior wall	V_4
	V_5	Fifth intercostal space, anterior axillary line, to heart	Lateral wall	V_5
	V_6	Fifth intercostal space, mid-axillary line, to heart	Lateral wall	V_6

Diagnostic Tests

Comparing two-dimensional and M-mode echocardiography

M-mode echocardiography sends a single ultrasonic beam to the heart, producing a columnar view of cardiac structures. In two-dimensional echocardiography, an arched ultrasonic beam sent to the heart produces a fan-shaped cross-sectional image of cardiac structures, showing how the structures relate spatially.

This illustration shows how M-mode and two-dimensional echocardiography differ. The shaded areas beneath the transducer identify the cardiac structures that intercept and reflect the transducer's ultrasonic waves. In M-mode echocardiography, this area is columnar, and echo tracings are plotted against time. In two-dimensional echocardiography, the scanning area comprises an arc of 30° and appears as a real-time TV display.

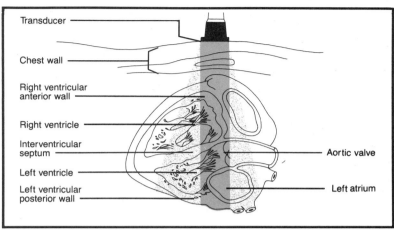

Echocardiography

This noninvasive imaging technique records ultrasonic waves reflected from the patient's heart, visualizing heart size and shape, myocardial wall thickness and motion, and cardiac valve structure and function. It also helps evaluate overall left ventricular function, detects some MI complications, and can determine mitral valve prolapse; mitral, tricuspid, or pulmonic valve insufficiency; cardiac tamponade; pericardial diseases; cardiac tumors; prosthetic valve function; subvalvular stenosis; ventricular aneurysms; cardiomyopathies; and congenital abnormalities.

To create an "acoustic window," conductive jelly is applied to the patient's chest at the third or fourth intercostal space just left of the sternum. A transducer placed on the patient's chest sends ultrasound waves to the heart; the waves reflect back to the transducer, which reabsorbs them. These ultrasonic echoes, translated into electrical signals, appear on an oscilloscope for viewing and recording.

Nursing considerations. Reassure the patient that echocardiograms don't cause pain or pose any risks.

Positron emission tomography (PET)

This noninvasive scanning method permits viewing of body organs and structures. Unlike other imaging methods, such as CT and MRI, which show organ structure, PET reveals physiologic activity. Used mainly for diagnosing central nervous system disorders, PET can also provide information about myocardial perfusion, myocardial metabolism of fatty acids and sugars, amino acid uptake, and infarction size. The patient receives an injection of a radioactive substance that decays gradually. A camera with special phototubes and multiple lenses records the amount of radioactive decay and transmits this information to a computer, which converts this information to a visual image for interpretation.

Radionuclide imaging

These noninvasive methods investigate coronary artery blood flow and ventricular contraction, using special cameras, computers, and intravenously injected radiopharmaceutical drugs. As the drugs decay, giving off gamma rays, a computerized scintillation camera takes pictures. Fed into the computer, these pictures produce an image that shows the drugs' concentration in a particular area. The doctor can then distinguish healthy tissue from damaged or diseased tissue by examining the serial pictures and can identify heart regions that don't contract normally. The most common radionuclide-imaging methods include thallium scanning, 99m technetium pyrophosphate scanning, and radionuclide venography.

Thallium scanning

Also known as "cold spot" imaging, this test evaluates myocardial blood flow and myocardial cell status. Thallium scanning can determine areas of ischemic myocardium and infarcted tissue and can evaluate coronary artery and ventricular function and pericardial effusion. Thallium imaging can also detect an MI in its first few hours.

Continued on page 18

Diagnostic Tests

Magnetic resonance imaging (MRI)

Also known as nuclear magnetic resonance (NMR), this diagnostic method yields high-resolution, tomographic, three-dimensional images of body structures. MRI permits visualization of valve leaflets and structures, pericardial abnormalities and processes, ventricular hypertrophy, cardiac neoplasm, infarcted tissue, anatomical malformations, and structural deformities. This test takes advantage of certain body nuclei that magnetically align, and then fall out of alignment, after radioactive transmission. The MRI scanner records the signals the nuclei emit as they realign in a process called precession, and then translates the signals into detailed pictures of body structures. The resulting images show tissue characteristics without lung or bone interference.

Compared to CT scanning, MRI yields an image with higher resolution, better contrast, and clearer delineation of detail. And because the technique doesn't emit radiation, serial MRI studies pose no danger to pregnant women and children. However, MRI takes a relatively long time to produce an image, and may not prove feasible for diagnosing diseases affecting several body systems.

Nursing considerations. Warn the patient that he'll remain completely enclosed in the MRI scanner during the 3-to-5 minute test. Have him remove all jewelry and other metallic objects before testing. A patient with an internal surgical clip, scalp vein needle, pacemaker, gold fillings, heart valve prosthesis, or other fixed metallic objects in or on his body can't undergo an MRI test. If the patient has an I.V. line, make sure the indwelling catheter's non-metallic.

Radionuclide Imaging—*continued*

Thallium-201, a radioactive isotope that emits gamma rays, closely resembles potassium. When injected intravenously, the isotope enters healthy myocardial tissue rapidly, but enters areas with poor blood flow and damaged cells slowly. A camera counts the gamma rays and displays an image. Areas with heavy isotope uptake appear light, while areas with poor uptake, known as cold spots, look dark. Cold spots represent areas of reduced myocardial perfusion.

To distinguish normal from infarcted myocardial tissue, the doctor may order an exercise thallium scan followed by a resting perfusion scan. Ischemic myocardium appears as a reversible defect (the cold spot disappears). Infarcted myocardium shows up as a nonreversible defect (the cold spot remains).

Note: Recent studies show that a patient with a normal thallium scan but an abnormal coronary arteriogram doesn't risk another cardiac incident more than does a normal patient. However, a patient with an abnormal thallium scan but a normal arteriogram *does* have a higher risk of another acute coronary event.

Nursing considerations. Tell the patient to avoid heavy meals, cigarette smoking, and strenuous activity before the test. If your patient's scheduled for an exercise thallium scan, advise him to wear comfortable clothes or pajamas and snug-fitting shoes or slippers.

99ᵐ technetium pyrophosphate scanning

This test, also known as "hot-spot" imaging, or PYP scanning, helps diagnose acute myocardial injury by showing the location and size of newly damaged myocardial tissue. Especially useful for a patient who's had a transmural infarct, hot-spot imaging works best if done 12 hours to 6 days after symptoms arise. This technique also helps diagnose right ventricular infarctions; locate true posterior infarctions; assess trauma, ventricular aneurysm, and heart tumors; and detect myocardial damage from recent electric shock (such as defibrillation).

The patient receives an injection of 99ᵐ technetium pyrophosphate, a radioactive material absorbed by injured cells. A scintillation camera scans the heart and pictures damaged areas as hot spots or bright areas. A spot's size usually corresponds to the injury size.

Nursing considerations. No special pretest or post-test is needed.

Multiple gated acquisition (MUGA) scanning

The doctor may order this study, also called radionuclide ventriculography, blood pool imaging, gated heart study, or wall motion study, to:
- assess left ventricular function
- determine the extent of muscle impairment after MI
- judge the general level of cardiac function
- diagnose congestive heart failure
- evaluate a patient's response to therapy
- assess the extent of cardiac muscle damage.

Visualizing cardiac structures

Cardiac structures, as shown on a chest X-ray

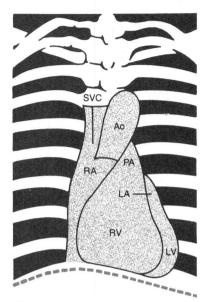

Key

SVC: Superior vena cava
RA: Right atrium
Ao: Aorta
PA: Pulmonary artery
RV: Right ventricle
LV: Left ventricle
LA: Left atrium

Diagnostic Tests

The patient receives an injection of a radiopharmaceutical that attaches to red blood cells and enters the circulatory system. A scintillation camera takes pictures of the heart and records the movement of these tagged blood cells and heart wall motion. These images, played like a motion picture, show blood flow through the heart. First-pass studies record radioactivity in the heart during one cardiac cycle. MUGA scanning records several hundred cardiac cycles until a recurrent pattern of images shows the patient's heart wall motion. MUGA studies also permit comparison of end-diastolic and end-systolic counts of tagged red blood cells. This permits the doctor to estimate ejection fraction—a good index of overall ventricular strength. MUGA's proven safe for patients too unstable to risk coronary angiography; for example, those with congestive heart failure or a recent MI. (However, frequent extrasystoles or irregular rhythms may skew test results or impair the procedure.)

Nursing considerations. Encourage the patient scheduled for MUGA to reduce his stress and activity levels and to avoid heavy meals before the test. If he'll exercise during the test, tell him to wear comfortable clothing and snug-fitting shoes.

Chest X-ray

The doctor will order a chest X-ray to detect cardiac enlargement, pulmonary congestion, pleural effusion, and calcium deposits in or on the heart. A chest X-ray also shows placement of a pacemaker, hemodynamic monitoring lines, and tracheal tubes. *Note:* Although a chest X-ray can reveal a cardiac problem, it can't prove its absence. Therefore, you can't evaluate cardiac function solely with an X-ray. Also, clinical signs may reflect your patient's condition 24 to 48 hours before they appear on X-ray.

Cardiac series

Largely superceded by echocardiography, the cardiac series studies heart motion through fluoroscopy. It assesses structural abnormalities of heart chambers, detects aortic and mitral valve calcification and abnormalities of the aortic arch and esophageal contours, and evaluates prosthetic valve function.

Pulse wave tracings

Risk-free and painless, these studies graphically record low-frequency vibrations from the carotid artery or jugular vein that reflect the heart's pulsations during systole and diastole. When compared with findings from other tests, such as EKGs and phonocardiograms, pulse wave tracings provide specific diagnostic information. For example, jugular vein tracings help identify tricuspid valve disorders and right-sided heart failure causing increased right atrial pressure. Carotid artery pulse tracings can detect aortic valve disease, idiopathic hypertrophic subaortic stenosis, left ventricular failure, and hypertension. An apexcardiogram (precordial pulsation tracing) can help identify heart sounds and ventricular enlargement.

Nursing considerations. Reassure the patient that the test won't cause discomfort. Note that a patient scheduled for a pulse wave tracing will probably also undergo phonocardiography or EKG studies.

Diagnostic Tests

Right and left heart catheterization

Both right and left heart catheterization use the antecubital and femoral vessels. For right heart catheterization, the catheter's inserted through veins to the superior or inferior vena cava and to the right atrium and ventricle. For left heart catheterization, the catheter's inserted through arteries to the aorta and into the coronary artery orifices and/or left ventricle.

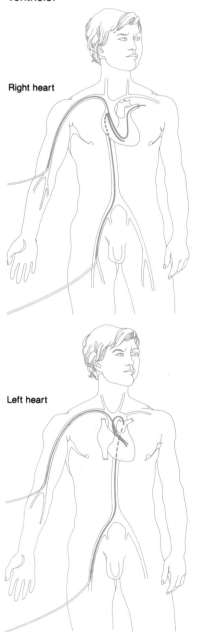

Right heart

Left heart

Cardiac catheterization and coronary angiography

This common invasive test for diagnosing heart disease uses a catheter threaded through an artery and vein into the heart to determine a coronary lesion's size and location, to evaluate left ventricular function, and to measure heart pressures. During the procedure, the doctor can also perform percutaneous transluminal coronary angioplasty (PTCA), inject intracoronary streptokinase, or evaluate the patient's left ventricular function prior to coronary artery bypass graft (CABG) surgery.

By catheterizing the right heart, the doctor can assess right ventricular function; determine tricuspid and pulmonic valve patency; detect intracardiac shunts; diagnose pulmonary hypertension; and measure cardiac output. With left heart catheterization, the doctor can assess left ventricular function and determine mitral and aortic valve patency. Using angiography, he can observe the heart's pumping performance, detect CAD, and identify vessels in need of bypass grafting.

The catheter enters the body through either the brachial artery (Sones procedure) or the femoral artery (Judkins procedure). The doctor then passes the catheter to the aortic root—the location of the coronary artery openings. In right heart catheterization, he passes a multilumen catheter through the superior or inferior vena cava into the right atrium, to the right ventricle, and into the pulmonary artery. A fluoroscope monitors the catheter's progress, while other instruments measure and record pressures within each chamber. The doctor can draw blood samples from the chambers for oxygen content and saturation analysis. Cardiac output can also be calculated using the thermodilution technique. Once the catheter reaches the pulmonary artery, pulmonary artery and pulmonary capillary wedge pressures can be obtained.

In left heart catheterization, the doctor threads a single-lumen catheter into the selected artery either percutaneously or via an arteriotomy. He then advances the catheter into the aorta, through the aortic valve and into the left ventricle. In a procedure known as ventriculography, he injects a radiopaque dye, which permits filming (cineangiography) of heart activity. The film shows how well the left ventricle flushes out the dye and identifies any ventricular areas that don't pump properly.

Next, the doctor removes the single-lumen catheter and inserts two specially shaped catheters to study the left and right coronary arteries. He then injects a second dye, and films the dye's flow through the arteries. This procedure identifies such problems as a narrowed or blocked coronary artery.

During catheterization, which takes about 2 hours, monitors continuously track the patient's heart rate and rhythm. After the procedure, pressure must be applied to the insertion site to stop the bleeding. A patient who's had the femoral approach must stay flat for 6 to 12 hours after catheterization to minimize the bleeding risk. *Continued on page 22*

Diagnostic Tests

Cardiac catheterization complications

Cardiac catheterization imposes more patient risk than most other diagnostic tests. Although such complications occur infrequently, they're potentially life-threatening. Cardiac catheterization requires careful observation during the procedure. Keep in mind that some complications arise in *both* left-heart and right-heart catheterization; others result only from catheterization of one side. In either case, notify the doctor promptly and carefully document the complications and their treatment.

Complication/Possible cause	Signs and symptoms
LEFT- OR RIGHT-SIDE CATHETERIZATION	
Hematoma or blood loss at insertion site • Bleeding at insertion site from vein or artery damage	Bloody dressing; limb swelling or increased girth; decreased blood pressure; tachycardia
Dysrhythmias • Cardiac tissue irritated by catheter	Irregular heartbeat; palpitations; ventricular tachycardia; ventricular fibrillation
Myocardial infarction • Emotional stress induced by procedure • Plaque dislodged by catheter tip that travels to a coronary artery (left-side catheterization only) • Occlusion of diseased artery by dye or catheter during procedure	Chest pain, possibly radiating to left arm, back, and/or jaw; cardiac dysrhythmias; diaphoresis, restlessness, and/or anxiety; thready pulse; nausea and vomiting
Reaction to contrast medium • Allergy to iodine	Fever; agitation; hives, itching; difficulty breathing
Hypovolemia • Diuresis from angiography contrast medium	Hypotension; tachycardia; pallor; diaphoresis
Infection (systemic) • Poor aseptic technique • Catheter contamination	Fever; tachycardia; chills and tremors; unstable blood pressure
Infection at insertion site • Poor aseptic technique	Swelling, warmth, redness, and soreness at insertion site; purulent discharge at insertion site
Cardiac tamponade • Perforation of heart wall by catheter	Dysrhythmias; tachycardia; decreased blood pressure; chest pain; diaphoresis; cyanosis; distant heart sounds
Pulmonary edema • Excessive fluid administration	Early stage: tachycardia, tachypnea, dependent crackles, diastolic (S_3) gallop. Acute stage: dyspnea; rapid, noisy respirations; cough with frothy, blood-tinged sputum; cyanosis with cold, clammy skin; tachycardia; hypertension
LEFT-SIDE CATHETERIZATION	
Arterial embolus or thrombus in limb • Injury to artery during catheter insertion • Plaque dislodged from artery wall by catheter	Slow or faint pulse distal to insertion site; loss of warmth, sensation, and color in arm or leg distal to insertion site; sudden pain in extremity
Cerebrovascular accident (CVA) or transient ischemic attack (TIA) • Blood clot or plaque dislodged by catheter tip that travels to brain	Hemiplegia/paresis; aphasia; lethargy; confusion or decreased level of consciousness
RIGHT-SIDE CATHETERIZATION	
Thrombophlebitis • Vein damaged during catheter insertion	Vein is hard, sore, cordlike, and warm (vein may look like a red line above catheter insertion site); swelling at site
Pulmonary embolism • Dislodged blood clot	Shortness of breath; tachypnea; tachycardia; chest pain; pink-tinged sputum
Vagal response • Vagus nerve endings irritated in sinoatrial node, atrial muscle tissue, or atrioventricular junction	Hypotension; bradycardia; nausea

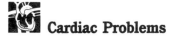

Diagnostic Tests

Coronary flow/perfusion evaluation

Using the same principles as DSA, coronary flow/perfusion evaluation can:

• assess blood flow through the coronary arteries

• investigate myocardial perfusion and myocardial anatomy

• determine the extent of coronary lesions.

A contrast medium injected into the coronary artery passes through the artery, entering cardiac tissue. A computer screen then displays a multicolored image, each color representing blood flow during subsequent cardiac cycles. The completed picture, called a Contrast Medium Appearance Picture, shows how long contrast medium takes to reach cardiac tissue.

Cardiac catheterization and coronary angiography—*continued*

Nursing considerations. Before catheterization: Take the patient's baseline vital signs. Note his anxiety and activity levels, and the presence and pattern of any chest pain. Document the presence of peripheral pulses, noting their intensity. Also identify any known allergies, particularly iodine or shellfish allergies, which suggest sensitivity to the radiopaque dye. Alert the doctor to any allergies or changes in the patient's condition.

Find out if the patient has signed the consent form. Make sure he understands why he's scheduled for catheterization. Explain that he won't receive general anesthesia but may be given a mild sedative during the procedure. Warn him that he may feel light-headed, warm, or nauseated for a few moments after the dye injection. Also tell him to expect some later discomfort at the insertion site, but assure him that he'll receive pain medication if necessary. Tell him to notify you immediately if he has any chest pain after the procedure.

Check with the doctor before withholding any medications. If your patient's scheduled for early morning catheterization, withhold foods and fluids after midnight of the preceding day.

After catheterization: Bleeding poses the most serious risk. If bleeding occurs, remove the pressure dressing and apply firm manual pressure. If the Judkins procedure was used, tell the patient to keep his leg straight for at least 6 to 8 hours. Elevate the head of the bed no more than 30°. If the Sones procedure was used, tell him to keep his arm straight for at least 3 hours. To immobilize the leg or arm, place a sandbag over it. For the first hour after catheterization, monitor the patient's vital signs every 15 minutes and inspect the dressing frequently for signs of bleeding. Also check the patient's skin color, temperature, and pulses distal to the insertion site. An absent or weak pulse may signify an embolus or another problem requiring immediate attention. Notify the doctor of any changes in peripheral pulses. If the patient's heart rhythm or vital signs change, or if he has chest pain (possible indications of dysrhythmias, angina, or MI), monitor the EKG closely and notify the doctor.

Your patient may complain of urinary urgency immediately after the procedure. Encourage him to drink fluids to flush out the dense radiopaque dye. Monitor urinary output, especially if his renal function's impaired. Also, check with the doctor about resuming any medications withheld before catheterization.

Digital subtraction angiography (DSA)

A refined version of coronary angiography, DSA combines angiography and computer processing to produce high-resolution images of cardiovascular structures. The images, converted to digital signals, with a number assigned to each color density from white to black, undergo a subtraction process. This eliminates interference and extraneous structures such as bone or soft tissue.

DSA helps evaluate coronary arterial flow, myocardial perfusion, and left ventricular function. Its advantages include:

• a reduced risk of complications associated with arterial puncture (because the contrast medium's injected into a vein)

• a clear view of arterial structures

• safer diagnosis of patients with heart failure, diabetes, and renal

Diagnostic Tests

Pulmonary artery catheter

Made of pliable radiopaque poly-vinylchloride, the pulmonary artery catheter may contain two to five lumens. Fluid-filled, the distal and proximal lumens monitor pressures. The thermistor connector lumen permits cardiac output measurement. The balloon inflation lumen, which inflates the catheter's balloon, allows pulmonary capillary wedge pressure measurement. The pacemaker wire lumen, which provides a port for pacemaker electrodes, also allows measurement of mixed venous oxygen saturation if an Opticath catheter's used.

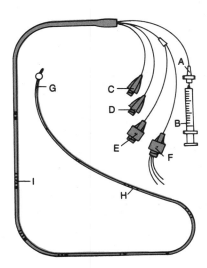

Key

A: Inflation lumen port

B: For balloon inflation with 1 to 1.5 ml of air

C: Distal lumen port

D: Proximal lumen port

E: Thermistor lumen port

F: Pacemaker wire lumen

G: Thermistor lumen opening

H: Proximal lumen opening

I: 10 cm markings

impairment (because the dilute, low-dose contrast medium won't depress cardiac and kidney function)
● outpatient use.

Nursing considerations. Prepare a patient for a DSA test as you would for cardiac catheterization. Urge him to stay as still as possible during the procedure. Also tell him that he'll have to hold his breath during the test to reduce movement that can mar image quality. Tell the patient to remain absolutely still during the test; even breathing or swallowing can impair image accuracy.

Left ventricular assessment. DSA can also evaluate left ventricular function and wall movement.

Hemodynamic monitoring

This technique assesses cardiac function and determines therapeutic effectiveness by measuring cardiac output, mixed venous blood, oxygen saturation, intracardiac pressures, or blood pressure. It also allows drawing of arterial blood. To use hemodynamic monitoring properly, you must fully understand the cardiac cycle.

Hemodynamic monitoring requires special pressurized tubing; a transducer to transform the blood's motion into an electrical impulse; and an oscilloscope with a screen to provide a readout, or waveform image, of the impulse. Follow your hospital's procedure for setting up, maintaining, and troubleshooting the equipment. (But remember, the monitor can't replace your clinical evaluation of the patient.)

We'll review several types of hemodynamic monitoring techniques, including those using the pulmonary artery catheter, left atrial pressure catheter, and arterial pressure catheter.

Equipment
Pulmonary artery (PA) catheter. This balloon-tipped, multilumen catheter, known as the Swan-Ganz catheter, permits measurement of intracardiac pressures. The doctor inserts the catheter into the patient's internal jugular or subclavian vein (in some cases, he'll use the basilar vein of the antecubital fossa). When the catheter reaches the right atrium, the doctor inflates the balloon to help float the catheter through the right ventricle into the pulmonary artery. This permits PCWP measurement through an opening at the catheter's tip. Deflated, the catheter rests in the pulmonary artery, allowing diastolic and systolic pulmonary artery pressure readings.

The PA catheter contains two to five lumens, the number of lumens determining which functions the catheter can perform. The distal lumen measures PA pressures when connected to a transducer and measures PCWP during balloon inflation. This lumen also permits drawing of mixed venous blood samples. The proximal (central venous pressure) lumen measures right atrial pressure; the ballon inflation lumen, as its name suggests, inflates the balloon at the distal tip of the catheter for PCWP measurement. The thermistor connector lumen contains temperature-sensitive wires, which feed information into a computer for cardiac output calculation. The

Continued on page 24

Diagnostic Tests

Viewing a typical arterial blood pressure waveform

The arterial waveform (shown in the illustration below) allows you to visualize the patient's cardiac cycle. The dicrotic notch represents aortic valve closure, which signals systole's end and diastole's start.

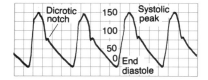

Intracardiac pressures

This flowchart illustrates the intracardiac pressures and their relationship to the cardiopulmonary systems.

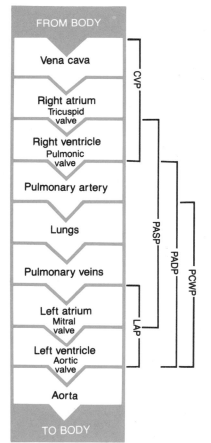

pacemaker wire lumen provides a port for pacemaker electrodes and measures mixed venous oxygen saturation (with Opticath catheter use).

Arterial blood pressure catheter. The doctor inserts this into the radial or femoral artery to measure blood pressure or obtain samples of arterial blood for diagnostic tests, such as ABGs. A transducer transforms the flow of blood during systole and diastole into a waveform, which then appears on an oscilloscope.

Left atrial pressure catheter. Inserted into the left atrium during open heart surgery, this catheter measures left heart pressure.

Intracardiac pressures

To understand intracardiac pressures measured by hemodynamic monitoring catheters, picture the heart and vascular system as a continuous loop with constantly changing pressure gradients that keep the blood moving. Hemodynamic monitoring records the gradients within the vessels and heart chambers.

Central venous pressure (CVP) or right atrial pressure (RAP). In diastole, the tricuspid valve opens and the right atrium and right ventricle merge (see illustration on page 25). The CVP or RAP shows right ventricular, or right heart, function and end-diastolic pressure. A transducer (as with a PA catheter) or a water-filled manometer measures RAP. Normal mean pressure ranges from 1 to 6 mm Hg (2 to 8 cm H_2O). (To convert mm Hg to cm H_2O, multiply the mm Hg by 1.34). Increased RAP may signal right ventricular failure, volume overload, tricuspid valve stenosis or regurgitation, constrictive pericarditis, pulmonary hypertension, cardiac tamponade, or right ventricular infarction. Decreased RAP suggests reduced circulating blood volume.

Right ventricular pressure (RVP). Generally, the doctor measures RVP only when initially inserting a PA catheter. RV systolic pressure normally equals pulmonary artery systolic pressure; RV end-diastolic pressure, which reflects RV function, equals RA pressure. Normal systolic pressure ranges from 15 to 25 mm Hg; normal diastolic pressure, from 0 to 8 mm Hg. RV pressures rise in mitral stenosis or insufficiency, pulmonary disease, hypoxemia, constrictive pericarditis, chronic congestive heart failure, atrial and ventricular septal defects, and patent ductus arteriosus.

Pulmonary artery pressures (PAPs). During systole, when the pulmonic valve opens and the mitral valve closes, the right ventricle and the left atrium act as a single chamber (see illustration on page 25). Pulmonary artery systolic pressure (PASP) shows right ventricular function and pulmonary circulation pressures. During diastole, the pulmonic valve closes and the mitral valve opens, allowing the pulmonary artery and the left ventricle to act as one (see illustration on page 25). Pulmonary artery diastolic pressure (PADP) reflects left heart pressures, specifically left ventricular end-diastolic pressure (LVEDP), in a patient without significant pulmonary disease. Systolic pressure normally ranges from 15 to 25 mm Hg; diastolic pressure, 8 to 15 mm Hg. The mean pressure usually ranges from 10 to 20 mm Hg. PADP rises in left ventricular (LV) failure, increased pulmonary blood flow (left or right shunting,

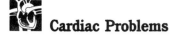

Diagnostic Tests

Measuring heart chamber pressures

Right atrial pressure (RAP)

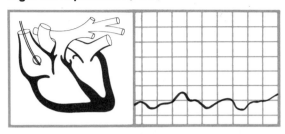

As the pulmonary artery catheter passes through the right heart chambers to its wedge position, it produces distinctive waveforms showing the catheter's position on the oscilloscope screen. As the tip reaches the right atrium from the superior vena cava, the waveform looks like this.

Pulmonary artery pressure (PAP)

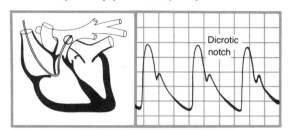

The waveform above indicates that the balloon has floated the catheter tip through the pulmonic valve into the pulmonary artery. The dicrotic notch reflects pulmonic valve closure.

Right ventricular pressure (RVP)

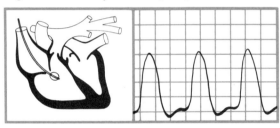

When the catheter tip reaches the right ventricle, the waveform looks like this.

Pulmonary capillary wedge pressure (PCWP)

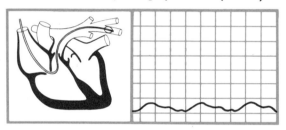

Blood flow in the pulmonary artery then carries the catheter balloon into a smaller pulmonary artery branch. When the vessel becomes too narrow for the balloon to pass through, the balloon wedges there. A waveform like this then appears.

as in atrial or ventricular septal defects), and in any condition causing increased pulmonary arteriolar resistance (such as pulmonary hypertension, volume overload, mitral stenosis, or hypoxia).

PCWP. To obtain PCWP, inflate the PA catheter balloon and wedge it in a pulmonary artery branch. The heart momentarily relaxes during diastole as it fills with blood from the pulmonary veins. This permits the pulmonary vasculature, left atrium, and left ventricle to act as a single chamber with identical pressures. Thus, PCWP reflects left atrial and LV pressures, unless the patient has mitral stenosis (see illustration above). Changes in PAP and PCWP reflect changes in LV filling pressure. The mean pressure normally ranges from 6 to 12 mm Hg. *Important:* Make sure the balloon's totally deflated (except when taking a PAWP reading). Prolonged wedging may cause pulmonary infarction. PCWP rises in LV failure, mitral stenosis or insufficiency, and pericardial tamponade. PCWP decreases in hypovolemia.

Left atrial pressure (LAP). This value reflects left ventricular end-diastolic pressure (LVEDP) in a patient without mitral valve disease. Mean LAP normally ranges from 6 to 12 mm Hg.

Continued on page 26

Diagnostic Tests

Hemodynamic Monitoring—*continued*

Other hemodynamic tests.
A fiberoptic oximeter thermodilution pulmonary artery catheter (Opticath) can measure mixed venous oxygen saturation (SVo_2). This procedure helps predict changes in cardiac output and determine treatment of a patient with heart failure or CAD.

Cardiac output measurement. Cardiac output indicates the amount of blood ejected by the heart each minute. In normal adults, cardiac output ranges from 4 to 8 liters. However, this amount varies with a patient's weight, height, and body surface area. Adjusting the cardiac output to the patient's size yields a measurement called the cardiac index. Cardiac output's determined from injection of a solution of known temperature and volume through a PA catheter's proximal lumen. This solution mixes with the blood of the superior vena cava or right atrium (depending on the location of the PA catheter). When this blood flows past a thermistor embedded in the PA catheter's distal end, the thermistor detects the temperature of the blood and solution and relays a signal to a computer. After analyzing this information, the computer displays the patient's cardiac output on a screen. (For more information on cardiac output, see Chapter 5.)

Self Test

1. Key signs and symptoms vital to early recognition of a cardiac problem may include all of the following, except:
a. cyanosis   **b.** edema   **c.** dyspnea   **d.** syncope

2. Which of the following heart sounds occurs most commonly in congestive heart failure?
a. S_1 **b.** S_2 **c.** S_3 **d.** S_4

3. To assess a patient with a cardiac problem, inspect his:
a. level of consciousness   **b.** skin and mucous membranes
c. jugular veins and carotid arteries   **d.** all of the above

4. If your patient's pulmonary capillary wedge pressure (PCWP) decreases, suspect:
a. left ventricular failure   **b.** mitral stenosis   **c.** cardiac tamponade
d. hypovolemia

5. On a 12-lead EKG strip, which of the following would you expect to see in lead V_1?
a. tall R wave   **b.** small R wave   **c.** tall Q wave   **d.** small Q wave

6. Which of the tests below helps determine myocardial cell viability and perfusion?
a. thallium scan   **b.** 99 technetium pyrophosphate scan
c. MUGA scan   **d.** magnetic resonance imaging (MRI)

Answers (page number shows where answer appears in text)

1. **a** (page 4)   2. **c** (page 11)   3. **d** (pages 6-7)   4. **d** (page 25)
5. **b** (page 15)   6. **a** (page 17)

Coronary Artery Disease/Angina: Coronary Artery Blockage

Coauthors **Sharon and John VanRiper** work at the University of Michigan Medical Center in Ann Arbor. Sharon, assistant head nurse, received her MS from the University. John, a surgical intensive care nurse, received his BSN from Wayne State University in Detroit.

In this section (which includes Chapters 3 through 7), we'll discuss the abnormalities of cardiac function and structure listed below:

• *interference in coronary artery blood flow:* coronary artery disease (angina pectoris and myocardial infarction)
• *pump failure or dysfunction:* heart failure and cardiomyopathies
• *inflammatory conditions:* pericarditis, endocarditis, and myocarditis
• *inadequate valve functioning:* stenosis and valve insufficiency.

But first, here's a quick review of cardiac anatomy (see illustration below) and physiology, particularly the heart's blood vessels.

Continued on page 28

Inside the normal heart

The right atrium lies in front and to the right of the smaller but thicker-walled left atrium. An interatrial septum separates the atria. The right atrium receives blood from the superior and inferior venae cavae. The left atrium receives blood from the four pulmonary veins. The right ventricle, forming the largest part of the heart's sternocostal surface and inferior border, sits behind the sternum. The left ventricle forms the heart's apex and most of its left border and diaphragmatic surface.

The tricuspid valve, with its three triangular cusps (leaflets), guards the right atrioventricular orifice. The cusps attach to the chordae tendineae by the papillary muscles in the right ventricle. The bicuspid, or mitral, valve protects the left atrioventricular opening. Its two cusps join the papillary muscles by chordae tendineae in the left ventricle. The two semilunar valves (the pulmonic and aortic valves) and their three cusps guard the aorta and the pulmonary artery orifices.

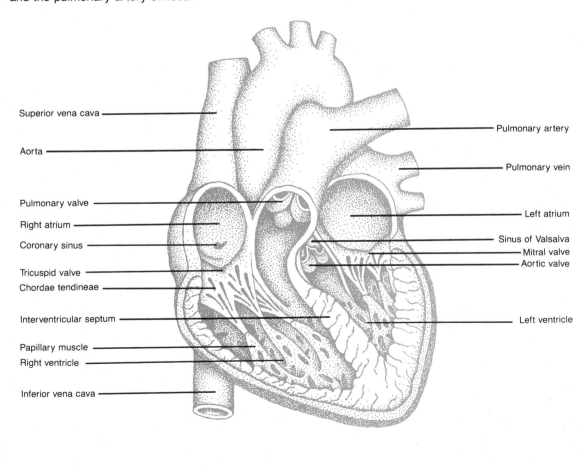

Coronary Artery Disease/Angina

Continued

Coronary arteries. The right and left coronary arteries originate from the aorta at the ostia, situated above the cusps of the aortic valve (the sinus of Valsalva). Lying free in epicardial fat, the left main coronary artery measures a few millimeters to a few centimeters long. This artery branches, forming the left anterior descending (LAD) and circumflex arteries. The LAD artery, descending toward the heart's apex, continues from the left main coronary artery more directly and serves as the origin for the diagonal arteries and septal perforators. The LAD artery and its branches supply blood to the anterior wall of the left ventricle, the anterior intraventricular septum, and the bundle branches.

The circumflex artery, circling the left ventricle and ending on its posterior surface, provides blood to the left ventricle's lateral and posterior portions. The obtuse marginal artery arises from the circumflex artery.

The right coronary artery fills the groove between the atria and the ventricles, giving rise to the acute marginal artery. It ends as the posterior descending artery.

The right coronary artery sends blood to the sinus and atrioventricular nodes as well as to the right atrium and ventricle. The posterior descending artery supplies the left ventricle's posterior and inferior wall and the right ventricle's posterior portion.

Coronary artery anastomoses. The heart's vessels communicate, both on the internal and external surfaces and throughout cardiac tissue. Epicardial anastomoses over the ventricles serve as important avenues for collateral circulation. Their structure and arterial pressure determine whether coronary anastomoses can carry collateral circulation. Adequate pressure ensures a gradient sufficient to permit blood flow.

Arterial supply. Coronary arteries can be epicardial or perforating. The former lie throughout the heart's surface; the latter penetrate ventricular walls, supplying the deep muscle layers. Coronary arteries receive blood flow primarily during diastole.

Coronary artery flow. A coronary artery's blood flow depends on its anatomy and chamber pressure, as well as certain metabolic factors. Because the coronary ostia sit near the aortic valve, they become partially occluded during systole when the valve leaflets open. During diastole, the aortic valve closes, leaving the ostia unobstructed. This permits filling and flow.

Chamber pressure. The coronary arteries arise on the epicardial surface, with some branches penetrating deeply into the myocardium. During systole, contraction impedes arterial blood flow. During diastolic relaxation, coronary arterial pressure drops, allowing increased perfusion. If intracardiac diastolic pressure increases—as in heart failure—coronary perfusion could suffer. If diastole shortens, as it does when heart rate quickens, blood flow to heart tissue decreases.

Metabolic factors. Physiologic and pharmacologic factors that influence the metabolic regulation of coronary circulation include neurohormonal responses, autoregulatory receptor activity, ischemia, and certain drugs.

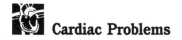
Coronary Artery Disease/Angina

The coronary arteries

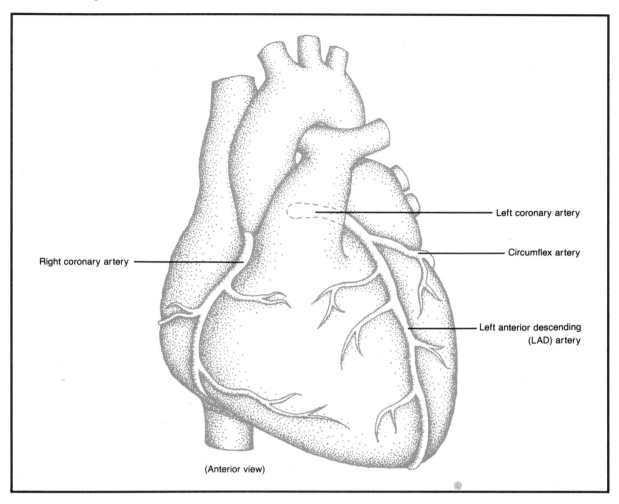

Left coronary artery

Circumflex artery

Right coronary artery

Left anterior descending (LAD) artery

(Anterior view)

Alpha and beta receptors affect coronary vessel resistance via catecholamines. Located in the peripheral vasculature, alpha receptors constrict blood vessels. Beta receptors in the heart and lungs respond to stimulation by increasing heart rate, respiration, myocardial oxygen uptake, and muscle contractility.

Norepinephrine briefly reduces coronary vascular resistance, then increases it for a prolonged time. These changes move blood into the body's central compartment, elevating blood pressure.

When aortic baroreceptors sense a blood pressure drop, they speed the heart rate and reduce coronary vascular resistance. This dual effect helps increase blood pressure while maintaining adequate blood flow to the heart. Should blood pressure drop below 60 or 70 mm Hg, the vascular bed dilates fully, making perfusion dependent on pressure alone. If perfusion pressure stays low, collateral blood flow slows—a particular threat to the myocardial infarction (MI) patient because loss of collateral flow could enlarge infarct size.

If coronary artery lesions develop, the artery's distal portion may already have dilated fully. Such an artery lacks reserve capacity for further dilation in the face of continued oxygen needs. But in normal vessels, higher oxygen demands cause dilation, which decreases perfusion pressure to distal diseased vessels. As perfusion

Continued on page 30

Coronary Artery Disease/Angina

Atherosclerosis stages

As shown in the illustration below, atherosclerosis starts with an injury to the intimal layer of the arterial wall (or some other pathologic event). This makes the wall permeable to circulating lipoproteins.

Lipoproteins invade smooth muscle cells in the intimal layer, forming a fatty streak—a nonobstructive lesion.

Eventually a fibrous plaque develops, impeding blood flow through the artery. Plaques contain lipoprotein-filled smooth muscle cells, collagen, and muscle fibers.

In the final stage of the atherosclerotic process, a complicated lesion appears, marked by calcification or rupture of the fibrous plaque. Thrombosis can occur, with near-total occlusion of the arterial lumen.

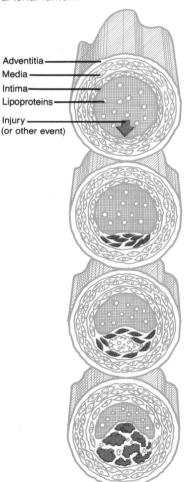

Adventitia
Media
Intima
Lipoproteins
Injury
(or other event)

Continued

pressure drops, blood flow decreases, causing yet more ischemic damage—a phenomenon called coronary steal.

Coronary circulation also suffers in hypoxia, which profoundly dilates vessels. The dilatory effect may stem from accumulation of adenosine within the cells. Prostaglandins, kinins, and potassium may also change vascular tone during hypoxia.

Calcium channel blockers dilate coronary arteries directly. In a patient with myocardial ischemia, nitrates redistribute blood through collateral circulation rather than dilating vessels. Alpha-adrenergic agents such as norepinephrine constrict coronary arteries.

Coronary veins. Three venous systems drain the heart: thebesian veins, anterior cardiac veins, and the coronary sinus and its tributaries. The ostium of the coronary sinus channels blood from the coronary veins into the right atrium.

Coronary artery disease

You may know it as coronary heart disease or atherosclerotic heart disease. But regardless of the term you use, coronary artery disease (CAD) remains the most common cause of cardiac disease in adults and the leading cause of death in this country.

Characterized by narrowed or obstructed arterial lumina, CAD interferes with blood flow to heart muscle. Blood-starved myocardium can develop various ischemic diseases, including angina pectoris, MI, congestive heart failure, sudden cardiac death, and cardiac dysrhythmias. Collectively, these diseases make up CAD.

CAD most commonly results from atherosclerosis, a form of arteriosclerosis, or hardening of the arteries, found in vessels (such as the aorta and the coronary, illiac, and carotid arteries) that carry blood to the heart, brain, kidneys, arms, and legs. Coronary artery atherosclerosis occurs primarily in arteries on the heart's epicardial surface, sparing arteries within the heart wall.

Atherosclerosis evolves slowly, beginning in childhood and progressing throughout life. Signs and symptoms usually don't appear until middle age or later, when the heart's blood supply can't meet its needs.

As degenerative changes in the arterial wall occur, lipid deposits— plaques called atheromas—develop within and beneath the vessel's inner layer. Advanced atheromas contain smooth muscle cells and an underlying layer of lipid debris. Cholesterol derived from plasma low-density lipoproteins (LDLs) forms the major lipid constituent; triglycerides and phospholipids also appear in the lipid debris.

Atheromas usually arise in areas of turbulent blood flow, such as just beyond sites where vessel diameters decrease and where blood vessels fork. By increasing turbulence and decreasing diameter, elevated blood pressure favors plaque formation.

Why do coronary arteries show a particular vulnerability to atherosclerosis? Partly because the heart's overall oxygen supply de-

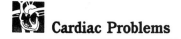

Coronary Artery Disease/Angina

creases from a near total lack of accessory blood supply. Atherosclerosis impedes coronary artery blood flow in these ways:
- plaques or thrombi obstruct the artery
- blood clots form around plaques
- hemorrhages form in damaged vessel walls beneath plaques
- hardened vessels can't dilate properly.

Tracing plaque formation. While no one knows exactly how atherosclerotic plaques form, scientists propose several theories. The most popular combines the insudation and encrustation theories. According to the *insudation theory,* high levels of total serum cholesterol or LDL cause deposits of cholesterol-rich lipoproteins to collect on the artery's intimal wall. These deposits penetrate the wall, resulting in a low-grade inflammatory response that produces edema in the intimal layer.

The *encrustation theory* holds that the inflammatory response triggers endothelial cell proliferation and increased platelet adhesion that gives rise to platelet aggregation. Platelets stimulate smooth muscle cells to multiply; cellular accumulation attracts fibrin and leukocytes. As the lesion enlarges, involving more of the intimal wall, the vascular obstruction grows. In some cases, hemorrhage occurs between the intimal and medial layers. In others, the lesion's center necrotizes. Many lesions calcify over time, creating a rough surface that promotes platelet aggregation and thrombus formation.

Other suggested mechanisms for plaque formation include the *monoclonal theory*, which proposes a "seeding" philosophy of plaque formation: Coronary lesions derive from a single smooth muscle cell that serves as the progenator for all proliferating cells.

The *lipogenic theory* relates the lesion's birth and progression to elevated LDL levels. As cholesterol infiltrates smooth muscle cells, the cells may necrotize, releasing lipids into extracellular spaces. Certain lipid substances stimulate smooth muscle cell proliferation while providing an environment conducive to connective tissue development.

The *endothelial injury theory* holds that coronary lesions result from intimal wall injury stemming from elevated LDL levels. Once injury occurs, platelets aggregate and release a factor that stimulates arterial smooth muscle cell proliferation on the intimal wall. If injury happens just once, the pathologic process can reverse itself. But repeated injury encourages progressive lesion development.

All four plaque formation theories suggest that the following factors characterize atherosclerosis:
- The artery's endothelial layer undergoes damage.
- LDL cholesterol infiltrates the intimal lining.
- Smooth muscle cells proliferate excessively.
- The process can't reverse itself.

While the pathogenesis of atherosclerosis remains unclear, no one disagrees as to the progressive pathologic changes the disease produces. First, a fatty streak—a smooth, yellowish lesion made up of lipid deposits—forms on the arterial wall. This small lesion can't obstruct blood flow, but it may develop into a raised fibrous

Continued on page 32

Coronary Artery Disease/Angina

Lipoprotein fractions

Chylomicrons, composed mainly of triglycerides derived from dietary fat, transport fats from the intestine to storage areas. Scientists haven't linked an elevated chylomicron level (Type I hyperlipoproteinemia) with CAD.

Very low-density lipoprotein (VLDL) consists of triglyceride. Manufactured in the liver and small intestine, VLDL transports glycerides. An elevated VLDL level (Type IV hyperlipoproteinemia) frequently appears in diabetic and obese patients and less commonly in young CAD patients.

Low-density lipoprotein (LDL), made primarily of cholesterol, results from VLDL breakdown. LDL has the greatest atherogenic potential. An elevated LDL level (Type II hyperlipoproteinemia) frequently goes hand in hand with an elevated VLDL level.

High-density lipoprotein (HDL), made of protein, probably helps remove excess cholesterol. Because people with high HDL levels have a lower CAD incidence, researchers believe HDL may protect against CAD.

Coronary artery disease—*continued*

plaque that *can*. In the final stage of the atherosclerotic process, a *complicated lesion*, or fibrous plaque, calcifies, ruptures, or thromboses.

Assessment

Because a patient can have coronary atherosclerosis for years without signs or symptoms, evaluating his risk factors can prove critical. So in addition to performing a standard cardiac assessment, identify any risk factors. One *major* risk factor combined with one or more *contributing* risk factors indicates a high CAD risk. The following review of risk factors will help.

Heredity. A family history of CAD or hyperlipidemia increases CAD risk.

Sex. More men develop CAD than women, and at a younger age; men age 40 to 55 have the highest risk. CAD ranks as the leading cause of death in men over age 40, and the chief cause of permanent disability in men under age 65. After about age 50, women become as likely as men to develop CAD, probably from hormonal changes that occur in both sexes. CAD takes a more complicated course in women.

Race. Black women of all ages and black men under age 45 have an increased incidence of hypertension, which increases the CAD risk.

Age. Despite a drop in serum cholesterol levels with advancing years, age remains a powerful CAD predictor. Studies show that the death rate from CAD increases with age.

The increasing odds for developing CAD as we age may merely stem from the aging process—or result from long-term exposure to risk factors. Another possible reason: as we age, high-density lipoprotein (HDL) can't keep pace with the influx of LDL, which favors cholesterol buildup in arteries. Essential hypertension, especially prevalent in the elderly, may also contribute to increased CAD risk.

Major controllable risk factors. Although your patient can't change his sex, race, or age, he *can* lower his CAD risk in other ways. Help your patient identify these factors by learning more about them.

High blood pressure. Consistently high blood pressure—either systolic or diastolic—poses the most important major CAD risk. Eventually, hypertension leads to atherosclerosis. The higher the pressure, the greater the chance of developing CAD. But even a modest pressure increase can lead to CAD in a patient with other risk factors. For example, as long as his blood pressure remains normal, a patient with an elevated serum cholesterol level may avoid CAD. But if he develops hypertension, he'll probably fall prey to CAD.

The chances of a hypertensive patient developing CAD exceed his combined risk for all other cardiovascular diseases, including stroke. Essential hypertension frequently affects middle-aged and elderly patients, blacks, heavy alcohol users, and oral contraceptive users. Many diabetic and gout patients also have hypertension. Consider any patient from these groups at risk for CAD.

While scientists can't fully explain how hypertension contributes to CAD, many suggest that increased blood pressure damages ar-

Coronary Artery Disease/Angina

CAD risk factors

MAJOR RISK FACTORS THAT CAN'T BE CHANGED
Heredity
Sex
Race
Age

MAJOR RISK FACTORS THAT CAN BE CHANGED
Cigarette smoking
High blood pressure
Blood cholesterol levels
Diabetes

CONTRIBUTING FACTORS
Obesity
Lack of exercise
Stress

terial linings. Atherosclerosis typically affects high-pressure vessels while sparing low-pressure vessels. In addition, gradual blood pressure escalation can lead to coronary vasoconstriction, left ventricular strain and eventual hypertrophy, and myocardial oxygen deficit.

Cigarette smoking. A man who smokes a pack of cigarettes daily stands more than twice the risk of developing CAD than a nonsmoker. If he smokes two or more packs a day, he's four times as likely to get the disease. Women smokers also increase their CAD risk. Regardless of sex, the more a patient smokes, the greater the risk. And a patient who has an MI runs a higher chance of dying within an hour of onset than does a nonsmoker—usually from dysrhythmia.

Smoking filter cigarettes won't reduce a smoker's CAD risk. But smoking cigars or pipes instead will lower his risk to that of a nonsmoker, as long as he doesn't inhale.

The good news: the effects of cigarette smoking seem reversible. Smokers who quit eventually return to the same risk level as people who've never smoked.

Scientists haven't found a single mechanism that explains smokers' increased CAD risk. But they suggest that smoking:
- constricts blood vessels (from nicotine inhalation)
- promotes thrombus formation by neutralizing the anticoagulant compound heparin
- stimulates platelet aggregation and the subsequent release of chemicals that cause vasospasm
- increases catecholamine levels, which speeds heart rate, elevates blood pressure, and irritates arterial linings
- promotes dysrhythmias, which diminish cardiac output and precipitate fatal rhythms in vulnerable patients
- decreases vital capacity
- lowers levels of vitamin C, necessary for cholesterol metabolism.

Serum cholesterol levels. The chance for CAD increases when serum cholesterol values exceed 200 mg/100 ml. Cholesterol's abrasive action damages the arteries, an effect exacerbated by high blood pressure. Cholesterol levels tend to increase, then decline, with age.

Serum cholesterol travels in lipoprotein complexes classified into fractions. Levels of total serum cholesterol depend on diet, HDL fraction, vessel pressures, genetic factors that govern the rate at which cholesterol leaves vessel walls, and clinically detectable cardiac disease. More men than women have abnormally high cholesterol levels.

Diabetes mellitus. Men with diabetes run twice the risk of CAD than nondiabetic men; diabetic women have a threefold greater risk. Researchers don't know why diabetes predisposes a patient to CAD, but they note that many diabetics have decreased HDL cholesterol levels, increased platelet adhesion, and other coagulation abnormalities. The high circulating levels of glucose in the poorly controlled diabetic may cause sugar deposition on arterial walls.

Continued on page 34

Coronary Artery Disease/Angina

Diagnosing CAD

If your patient lacks CAD symptoms such as chest pain, the doctor usually confirms CAD by identifying risk factors. For a symptomatic patient, he'll investigate the patient's history and the pattern of chest pain.

Diagnostic tests provide baseline data, help determine the extent of CAD, and help confirm the diagnosis. Expect the doctor to order a 12-lead EKG, chest X-ray, blood studies (such as enzyme levels, lipid profiles, and complete blood count tests), nuclear scans (such as thallium imaging, technetium 99 pyrophosphate, and blood pool imaging), echocardiogram, cardiac angiography, or cardiac catheterization. (Chapter 2 gives details on these tests.)

Coronary artery disease—*continued*

Contributing factors. These factors can contribute to the development of CAD risk factors.

Obesity. A patient with high blood pressure or elevated total cholesterol exacerbates his CAD risk if he's obese. When a hypertensive, obese patient loses weight, both his blood pressure and LDL levels drop.

An obese patient synthesizes and eliminates more cholesterol than does a patient with normal weight. HDL levels drop with obesity, probably from inactivity. By promoting glucose intolerance and adult onset diabetes mellitus, obesity further contributes to CAD.

Lack of exercise. Like obesity, inactivity (which frequently goes hand in hand with overeating and overweight) seems to accompany decreased HDL levels. Atherosclerosis progresses more rapidly in inactive than in active people.

Regular exercise increases HDL cholesterol levels, decreases plasma catecholamines, lowers resting heart rate, and may improve myocardial oxygenation—a benefit that may or may not decrease CAD risk.

Aerobic exercise improves oxygen extraction from the blood and only minimally elevates diastolic pressure. Anaerobic (isometric) exercise, on the other hand, dramatically increases blood pressure, which may lead to angina, heart failure, or dysrhythmias.

Researchers don't agree about how much or what types of exercise benefit the heart. Sudden death can follow vigorous exercise such as running, probably from ventricular fibrillation rather than cardiac disease.

Stress. By increasing levels of circulating catecholamines, stress may contribute to CAD; elevated catecholamine levels may increase blood pressure and myocardial oxygen consumption. Stress can also lead to overeating, fatigue, lack of exercise, and even dysrhythmias.

A patient with a so-called Type A personality runs twice the normal CAD risk in youth and middle age. Signs and symptoms of the Type A personality include chronic overreaction to stress; an exaggerated sense of urgency; excessive aggressiveness, competitiveness, and hostility; and compulsive striving for achievement.

Other risk factors. Other factors that may promote CAD include the following:

Left ventricular hypertrophy (LVH). A patient with LVH greatly risks CAD. Nearly half of the patients who die from cardiovascular disease first show signs of LVH. The condition stems from chronic hypertension, which forces the heart to pump harder against mounting pressure gradients. Like all muscles, the heart grows from the increased work load.

Oral contraceptive use. In most women, oral contraceptive use exacerbates the atherogenic process and, in particularly susceptible women, it also elevates blood pressure. Women smokers who use

Coronary Artery Disease/Angina

oral contraceptives increase their risk for CAD and MI. Some oral contraceptive users may also have increased blood coagulation (and possibly thrombosis), diseased blood vessels, and decreased HDL. Hormones in oral contraceptives affect blood cholesterol differently: estrogens may raise HDL levels, whereas progestins may lower them.

Gout. Twice as many men with gout get CAD as do their gout-free counterparts. The higher risk may result from increased blood lipids and blood pressure, obesity, and glucose intolerance—common gout effects.

Diet. A diet high in cholesterol and saturated fats may promote hypertension and raise blood cholesterol levels. High caffeine intake (more than six cups of coffee a day) may contribute to hypertension and dysrhythmias. On the other hand, moderate alcohol intake (one or two drinks a day) may reduce the risk of CAD. However, excessive alcohol consumption damages the myocardium.

Environmental factors. Some CAD research focuses on the effects of climate and the mineral content of drinking water. Studies suggest a higher CAD mortality rate in predominantly cold, snowy regions, whereas high altitude seems to reduce the incidence of CAD. While "hard" drinking water seems to confer some protection against CAD, researchers can't attribute this effect to specific trace elements.

Other CAD research investigates the role of autoimmune thyroid antibodies, angiotoxins, and prostaglandins.

Planning
Your care priorities for a CAD patient depend on the presence or absence of signs and symptoms. If he has signs and symptoms, make your first priority enhancing myocardial oxygenation and perfusion, to relieve chest pain and preserve myocardial tissue. If he lacks signs and symptoms—or if these have been stabilized—focus on identifying, minimizing, or correcting risk factors.

You'll probably find caring for the CAD patient a challenge. In addition to understanding the disease process, including its presentation and usual clinical progression, you'll have to assess your patient thoroughly and knowledgeably, paying close attention to any complaints of chest pain and indications of myocardial ischemia or heart failure. You'll also need to understand any diagnostic procedures the doctor may order, to explain them to the patient.

While your patient undergoes diagnostic tests to confirm the extent of CAD, educate and support the family to help them learn to live with the disease. You can play a vital role in helping your patient identify risk factors, develop strategies to eliminate them, or reduce their effects.

Nursing diagnoses. Before planning your care of a CAD patient, determine your nursing diagnoses by identifying his actual or potential problem and relating it to its origin or cause. Possible nursing diagnoses for a CAD patient include:

Continued on page 36

Coronary Artery Disease/Angina

Coronary artery disease—*continued*

- injury, potential for, (cardiac event); related to the presence of CAD risk factors
- comfort, alteration in, (chest pain); related to myocardial ischemia
- cardiac output, alteration in, (decreased); related to atherosclerosis
- knowledge deficit; related to disease
- noncompliance of treatment; related to inadequate health teaching
- coping, ineffective individual (or family); related to diagnosis
- family dynamics, alteration in; related to diagnosis
- anxiety, potential for; related to diagnosis
- health maintenance, alteration in; related to knowledge deficit, inadequate health teaching, or denial.

For an example of a nursing care plan for a CAD patient, see the box below. But remember to tailor your plan to the needs of your patient and his family or support persons. (*Note*: The generalized care plan below presents a sample listing of expected outcomes, nursing interventions, and discharge planning that may apply to your patient.)

Interventions

A CAD patient may require medical treatment such as diet, medication, exercise, and risk factor reduction. If drug therapy and risk factor reduction can't lower or eliminate his angina, he may need surgery; for example, percutaneous transluminal coronary angioplasty (PTCA) or coronary artery bypass grafting (CABG).

Percutaneous transluminal coronary angioplasty. Introduced as an alternative to bypass surgery, PTCA improves coronary blood flow by enlarging the diseased artery's lumen.

Compression of the lesion against the arterial wall by a pressurized balloon causes a local injury to that vessel. This triggers a healing process that promotes vessel dilation. Platelets aggregate and release prostacycline, a potent vasodilator, from the vessel wall. The platelets also release thromboxane (TxA_2), which aids in thrombus

Sample nursing care plan—CAD

Nursing diagnosis	Expected outcomes
Injury, potential for, (cardiac event); related to CAD risk factors.	The patient will: • Demonstrate an understanding of CAD risk factors. • Discuss the CAD risk factors affecting him. • Discuss ways to reduce risk factors. • Show knowledge of the reason for treatment. • Show knowledge of methods for preventing or reducing the chance of future cardiac injury or events.
Nursing interventions • Teach the patient about CAD risk factors. • Help the patient identify his risk factors. • Teach the patient strategies for interrupting or minimizing the effects of his risk factors. • Discuss the purpose of treatment, giving specific information about medications, diagnostic tests, diet, etc. • Discuss which CAD symptoms require medical attention. • Teach him how to modify his daily activities.	**Discharge planning** • Discuss with the patient and his family or support persons how to modify daily activities to help reduce risk factors. • Teach the patient when to seek medical attention. • Reinforce the need for CAD risk factor reduction and treatment. • Give resources and/or materials to support the patient's instructions. • Provide information about community-based support groups. • Teach the patient stress reduction techniques.

Coronary Artery Disease/Angina

Percutaneous transluminal coronary angioplasty

A balloon-tipped catheter (with balloon inflated) rests in a stenosed coronary artery. The close-ups below show first catheter placement in the stenotic artery, then how balloon inflation widens the vessel lumen.

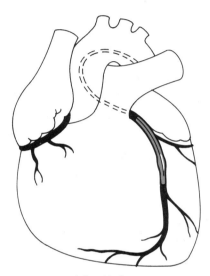

Inflated balloon

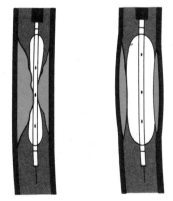

Catheter placement   Balloon inflation

formation. As a result, controlled injury occurs, with the healing process contributing to successful dilation of the arterial lumen.

Although doctors initially performed PTCA on patients with single-vessel disease, they may also use it to treat multivessel disease. PTCA best treats arteries with 50% to 95% blood flow reduction caused by noncalcified occlusions in the proximal LAD, left circumflex, or right coronary artery.

The doctor may perform emergency PTCA during acute episodes of unstable angina or in the first 4 to 6 hours after onset of chest pain in MI. When performing PTCA during an MI, the doctor may also administer streptokinase or urokinase via intracoronary infusion to promote thrombolysis and recanalization.

Procedure. The doctor guides a catheter through the ascending aorta and into the ostium of the right or left coronary artery. At this point, he performs angiography, then inserts a dilating catheter through the guiding catheter and into the artery's stenotic area. Continuous pressure monitoring reveals any blockage of the coronary artery ostium and permits measurement of the pressure gradient across the lesion.

Next, the doctor inflates the dilating catheter's balloon for 3 to 5 seconds with a half-and-half mixture of contrast medium and saline solution. He controls inflation with a pressure pump that lets him select pressures of 3 to 6.5 atmospheres. He then repeats angiography to evaluate the angioplasty's effect.

During or after the procedure, the doctor may order aspirin, nifedipine, heparin, dipyridamole, low molecular weight dextran, or nitroglycerin.

Complications. If PTCA fails, the patient will probably have to undergo CABG. And complications (for example, coronary artery occlusion, spasm, dissection, rupture, MI, hemorrhage, or hematoma) can also arise during the procedure, requiring immediate surgery.

Nursing care. Care for your patient as you would for a patient undergoing cardiac catheterization. Before PTCA, thoroughly assess his cardiovascular system. Also assess your patient's knowledge of PTCA, teaching him about the procedure, if necessary. Make sure he knows the potential risks or complications. Reinforce the doctor's explanation, reminding the patient that he must remain awake and assist with proper placement of the catheter by taking deep breaths when instructed. Also remind him that he may need CABG surgery if PTCA fails.

After PTCA, your patient will probably remain in the critical care unit for 24 hours, with arterial and femoral sheaths in the groin. The sheaths usually stay in place for 6 to 8 hours postprocedurally. You can use the arterial sheath for arterial pressure measurements. To keep it patent, employ a heparin flush solution. Be sure to check the catheter site frequently for bleeding and bruising. Remind your patient to keep his leg flat and to stay in bed. After sheath removal, apply a pressure dressing. Assess circulation frequently by checking for warmth and distal pulses.

Continued on page 38

Coronary Artery Disease/Angina

Laser angioplasty

Can lasers help revascularize coronary arteries? Researchers investigating laser angioplasty aim to vaporize the plaques and thrombi that block arteries in atherosclerosis. The technique may prove a useful adjunct to bypass (open-heart) surgery. Percutaneous transluminal laser angioplasty could also become available.

The doctor inserts a laser-containing catheter into the diseased artery. When the laser nears the problem area, the doctor switches it on and off in rapid bursts for a predetermined time period. Between bursts, he rotates the catheter, advancing it until he's completely opened the vessel. Repeat angiography documents vessel patency.

Experiments have yielded the best results in thrombi-obstructed arteries, but the technique can also remove calcified plaques. Limiting exposure time helps minimize intimal surface damage.

Laser angioplasty shows great potential. But before it can be used routinely, researchers must learn how heat generated during treatment affects red blood cells. They're also looking into effects of charred plaque remnants and gas emitted during vaporization, and hope to determine the proper intensity and exposure time for plaque destruction without damage to vessel walls. Finally, they must discover how to keep vessels patent after therapy.

Coronary artery disease—*continued*

Also watch for chest pain, shortness of breath, and changes in mental status, which may indicate a complication. Monitor vital signs carefully, paying particular attention to heart rate and rhythm. Check for increased ectopy and report any unusual findings to the doctor.

Before he's discharged, educate the patient about the medication he'll take and repeat any instructions about lowering his CAD risk.

Coronary artery bypass graft surgery. CABG surgery restores blood flow to an ischemic heart by bypassing the blockage in the coronary artery. The doctor uses a saphenous vein or internal mammary artery grafts to bypass the affected artery. Commonly bypassed arteries include the left main coronary artery, LAD, distal right coronary artery, posterior descending branch, and the marginal branch of the circumflex artery.

The following conditions may call for CABG surgery:
• chronic disabling angina pectoris unresponsive to medical therapy
• unstable or preinfarction angina unresponsive to medical therapy
• left main coronary artery stenosis that narrows more than half the artery's diameter
• three-vessel CAD
• continuing angina pectoris after MI.
Before recommending CABG, the doctor will also consider the patient's signs and symptoms, diagnostic test results, any operative risks, the patient's life quality before surgery, and the surgery's cost.

Procedure. While the surgical team prepares the patient for cardiopulmonary bypass, the doctor excises the graft and cannulates the inferior and superior venae cavae to divert blood to the heart-lung machine. Oxygenated blood returns to the arterial system through an arterial cannula positioned in the ascending aortic arch. (See page 39.)

After dilution and heparinization of the patient's blood to prevent clotting, and reduction of body temperature to 20°C to 28°C to conserve oxygen, the doctor injects a cold potassium blood cardioplegic (heart immobilizing) solution into the coronary arteries.

With blood flow diverted from the operative area and the patient properly prepared, the doctor next sews the grafts into place. He anastomoses the graft proximally to the ascending aorta, distally to the coronary arteries, beyond the occlusion site.

The surgical team then slowly weans the patient from the bypass machine. They may also insert pacemaker wires into his chest. After placing mediastinal drainage tubes and closing the sternum with wires to maintain stability, the doctor sutures the chest closed.

Complications. Complications during and after CABG surgery can cause debilitation or death. During surgery, an MI or cerebrovascular accident (CVA) may result from hypotension and/or hypoperfusion. After surgery, the patient may develop a dysrhythmia, bleeding disorders, blood gas disturbance, respiratory distress, wound infection, mental confusion, anxiety, and pain. The graft may become occluded and fail, CAD may progress, and the patient may have an MI.

Coronary Artery Disease/Angina

Bypass grafts

Bypassing a coronary artery occlusion, the doctor sutures a graft into place. Note that he's already bypassed two other occlusions.

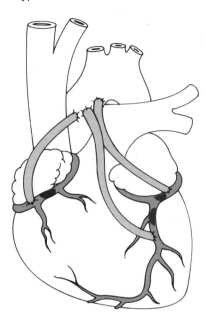

Nursing care. Thoroughly assess your patient's cardiovascular status before surgery, and educate him and his family or support persons. Explain the procedure and the possible risks and benefits. You might want to show the patient a drawing of the heart and coronary arteries or use a heart model, to demonstrate which arteries require bypass. If the doctor will use a saphenous vein graft, be sure the patient knows he'll have a long leg incision that may cause discomfort during the recovery period.

To prepare your patient for the immediate postoperative period, briefly explain the purpose of supportive equipment. Emphasize that the endotracheal tube may stay in place for 12 to 24 hours after surgery. Assure the patient that the health care team will anticipate his needs, even though the tube will prevent him from speaking.

After CABG, the patient will gradually increase his activities and independence. Many doctors start cardiac rehabilitation before the patient leaves the hospital. He'll probably stay at home for 6 to 8 weeks before resuming work. During this time, he'll gain strength and improve fitness through a prescribed activity program. Tell your patient to notify the doctor at once if pain or other angina symptoms recur.

Make sure the patient understands that CABG surgery won't cure CAD, only relieve the symptoms. He must still try to reduce any controllable risk factors. *Continued on page 40*

Maintaining blood flow during CABG surgery

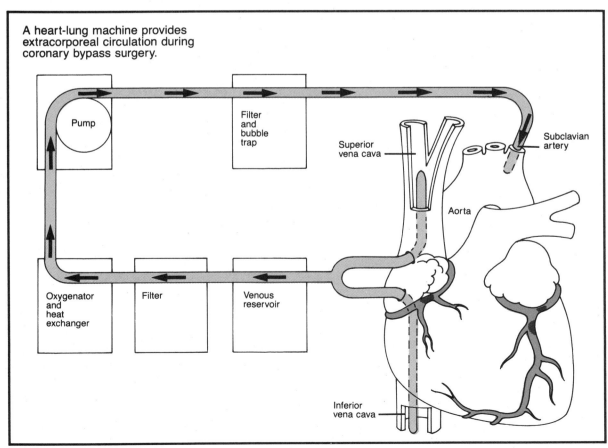

A heart-lung machine provides extracorporeal circulation during coronary bypass surgery.

Coronary Artery Disease/Angina

How prolonged bed rest and exercise affect the heart

Until recently, doctors treated cardiac patients conservatively, confining them to bed for weeks and prohibiting them from resuming active lives. But long bed rest can cause complications. For one thing, prolonged inactivity decreases work capacity, which in turn reduces maximal oxygen uptake. After 10 days of bed rest, blood volume decreases by 0.7 to 0.8 liters. When a hypovolemic patient becomes active again, he's likely to experience tachycardia and orthostatic hypotension. Because the decreased blood volume comes primarily from a drop in plasma rather than red cells, hypovolemia increases blood viscosity, predisposing the patient to thromboemboli. Negative nitrogen balance occurs, causing impaired wound healing. Prolonged bed rest also decreases skeletal muscle mass, muscular strength, and muscle efficiency, leading to oxygen debt. To repay the debt, the heart must pump more blood, straining an already weak myocardium.

In the 1970s, doctors began to encourage progressive and early ambulation, including exercise in cardiac rehabilitation. Patients treated this way had far fewer thromboembolic complications, reduced anxiety, and depression and resumed normal activities earlier.

Regular exercise also improves the cardiac patient's physical condition. Patients who exercise have lower resting pulse rates and blood pressures, which decrease myocardial oxygen use.

Although regular exercise clearly improves the patient's life quality, researchers can't prove that it prolongs life expectancy or prevents heart disease from progressing.

Coronary artery disease—*continued*

Cardiac rehabilitation. To help the CAD patient gain cardiovascular fitness while minimizing the chance of another cardiac event, the doctor may recommend a rehabilitation program. In addition to post-MI, CABG, and PTCA patients, those with angina pectoris, congestive heart failure, pacemakers, and valve replacements or disorders may also undergo rehabilitation. Such patients usually start rehabilitation as soon as their conditions stabilize.

All programs offer supervised exercise training and education while providing support for the patient and his family. Comprehensive programs have three phases, beginning with the acute inpatient setting and continuing indefinitely with long-term outpatient conditioning. An aerobic exercise program geared to the patient's disease, disabilities, and age includes supervised warm-up and cool-down periods. Graded exercise tests at set intervals help evaluate the patient's progress. Emergency equipment and trained personnel stay with the patient at all times. The rehabilitation team records the patient's progress and teaches him how to incorporate his exercises into his daily activities. Patients who've undergone cardiac rehabilitation programs report feelings of increased well-being, and many continue to exercise after graduating from the program.

Rehabilitation phases. Phase 1 takes place in the hospital. The patient participates in progressive self-care activities, ambulation, and exercise. He learns about the CAD process, risk factors, diet, and medication and finds out how to reduce his risk factors and modify his life-style to improve his health. He also learns to cope with any psychosocial problems.

Phase 2 begins when the patient leaves the hospital, and continues for about 8 weeks. Goals include gradually building strength, improving cardiovascular fitness, and gaining confidence. Most phase 2 programs offer educational programs and group social events to help the patient change his life-style. Some programs offer support groups to help spouses deal with their fears and problems, and may teach cardiopulmonary resuscitation to spouses and other family members.

Phase 3, designed to improve the patient's general physical condition, may continue indefinitely. Two or three weekly exercise sessions help the patient maintain his improved condition.

Evaluation

Base your evaluation of the CAD patient on his expected outcomes listed on your nursing care plan. To determine if he improved, ask yourself these questions:
- Does he understand CAD risk factors and how they apply to him?
- Can he discuss ways to reduce his risk factors?
- Does he understand the reason for his treatment?
- Does he know how to prevent or reduce his chance of future cardiac injury?

The answers to these questions will help you evaluate your patient's cardiac status and the effectiveness of his care. Keep in mind that these questions stem from the care plan shown on page 36. Your questions may differ.

Coronary Artery Disease/Angina

METS at a glance

Metabolic equivalents of a task (METs) measure an activity's work load on the cardiovascular and pulmonary systems. One MET equals 3.5 ml of oxygen consumption per kilogram of body weight per minute. The chart below shows how many METs various activities use. However, general fitness, fatigue, excitement, or emotional stress can alter MET values.

Keep this chart handy when educating your CAD patient about safe activity levels.

1 MET

Home activities
- Bed rest
- Sitting
- Eating
- Reading
- Sewing
- Watching television

Occupational activities
- No activity allowed

Exercise or sports activities
- No activity allowed

1 to 2 METs

Home activities
- Dressing
- Shaving
- Brushing teeth
- Washing at sink
- Making bed
- Desk work
- Driving car
- Playing cards
- Knitting

Occupational activities
- Typing (electric typewriter)

Exercise or sports activities
- Walking 1 mph (1.6 km/hr) on level ground

2 to 3 METs

Home activities
- Tub bathing
- Cooking
- Waxing floor
- Riding power lawn mower
- Playing piano

Occupational activities
- Driving small truck
- Using hand tools
- Typing (manual typewriter)
- Repairing car

Exercise or sports activities
- Walking 2 mph (3.2 km/hr) on level ground
- Bicycling 5 mph (8 km/hr) on level ground
- Playing billiards
- Fishing
- Bowling
- Golfing (with motor cart)
- Operating motorboat
- Horseback riding (at walk)

3 to 4 METs

Home activities
- General housework
- Cleaning windows
- Light gardening
- Pushing light power mower
- Sexual intercourse

Occupational activities
- Assembly-line work
- Driving large truck
- Bricklaying
- Plastering

Exercise or sports activities
- Walking 3 mph (4.8 km/hr)
- Bicycling 6 mph (9.7 km/hr)
- Sailing
- Golfing (pulling hand cart)
- Pitching horseshoes
- Archery
- Badminton (doubles)
- Horseback riding (at slow trot)
- Fly-fishing

4 to 5 METs

Home activities
- Heavy housework
- Heavy gardening
- Home repairs, including painting and light carpentry
- Raking leaves

Occupational activities
- Painting
- Masonry
- Paperhanging

Exercise or sports activities
- Calisthenics
- Table tennis
- Golfing (carrying bag)
- Tennis (doubles)
- Dancing
- Slow swimming

5 to 6 METs

Home activities
- Sawing softwood
- Digging garden
- Shoveling light loads

Occupational activities
- Using heavy tools
- Lifting 50 lbs

Exercise or sports activities
- Walking 4 mph (6.4 km/hr)
- Bicycling 10 mph (16.1 km/hr)
- Skating
- Fishing with waders
- Hiking
- Hunting
- Square dancing
- Horseback riding (at brisk trot)

6 to 7 METs

Home activities
- Shoveling snow
- Splitting wood
- Mowing lawn with hand mower

Occupational activities
- All activities listed previously

Exercise or sports activities
- Walking or jogging 5 mph (8 km/hr)
- Bicycling 11 mph (17.7 km/hr)
- Tennis (singles)
- Waterskiing
- Light downhill skiing

7 to 8 METs

Home activities
- Sawing hardwood

Occupational activities
- Digging ditches
- Lifting 80 pounds
- Moving heavy furniture

Exercise or sports activities
- Paddleball
- Touch football
- Swimming (backstroke)
- Basketball
- Ice hockey

8 to 9 METs

Home activities
- All activities listed previously

Occupational activities
- Lifting 100 pounds

Exercise or sports activities
- Running 5.5 mph (8.9 km/hr)
- Bicycling 13 mph (20.9 km/hr)
- Swimming (breaststroke)
- Handball (noncompetitive)
- Cross-country skiing
- Fencing

10 or more METs

Home activities
- All activities listed previously

Occupational activities
- All activities listed previously

Exercise or sports activities
- Running 6 mph (9.7 km/hr) or faster
- Handball (competitive)
- Squash (competitive)
- Gymnastics
- Football (contact)

Coronary Artery Disease/Angina

Angina characteristics

Quality
• Sensation of pressure or heavy weight on the chest
• Burning sensation
• Feeling of tightness
• Shortness of breath with feeling of constriction around the larynx or upper trachea
• Visceral quality (deep, heavy, squeezing, aching)
• Gradual increase in intensity followed by gradual fading

Location
• Over or near the sternum
• Anywhere between epigastrium and pharynx
• Occasionally limited to left shoulder and left arm
• Rarely limited to right arm
• Limited to lower jaw
• Lower cervical or upper throacic spine
• Left interscapular or suprascapular area

Duration
• 5 seconds to 30 minutes

Precipitating factors
• Exercise
• Raising arms above the head
• Cold temperatures
• Walking against the wind
• Walking after a large meal
• Emotional factors involved with physical exercise
• Fright, anger
• Sexual activity

Nitroglycerin relief
• Pain relief within 45 seconds to 5 minutes after taking nitroglycerin

Radiation
• Medial aspect of left arm
• Left shoulder
• Jaw
• Occasionally right arm

Adapted from Helfant, R.H., and Banka, V.S.: A Clinical and Angiographic Approach to Coronary Heart Disease, Philadelphia, F.A. Davis Co., 1978, p. 47.

Angina

When blood supply to the heart decreases, ischemic heart diseases may occur. Angina pectoris (known simply as angina) can result from ischemia. Paroxysmal chest pain from angina pectoris occurs when myocardial oxygen demand exceeds supply.

Atherosclerosis of the coronary arteries most commonly causes angina. Signs and symptoms usually result when one or more of the coronary arteries' three major branches are at least 75% occluded.

Less frequently, severe aortic stenosis or regurgitation, idiopathic hypertrophic subaortic stenosis, syphilitic stenosis of the coronary ostia, congenital anomalies of the coronary arteries, cardiomyop-

Angina: What goes wrong

Angina's episodic pain arises from myocardial hypoxia—oxygen deficiency. Hypoxia's causes include:
• decreased blood flow, resulting from atherosclerosis, thrombosis, embolism, or coronary artery spasm
• decreased oxygen carrying capacity of the blood, as in severe anemia
• increased myocardial work load (which intensifies the heart's oxygen needs), resulting from hypertension or aortic stenosis.

How angina develops

Stress activates the sympathetic nervous system, constricting blood vessels and increasing heart rate, contractility, and blood pressure. The result: ischemia and hypoxia that damage cardiac cells, white blood cells, and platelets. The injured cells release potassium, histamine, and serotonin, stimulating pain nerve endings. Meanwhile, metabolism switches from aerobic to anaerobic. The lactic acid produced further stimulates pain nerve endings.

The heart's sensory nerves stimulate nerves that synapse with sensory nerves from other body parts at the spinal cord's thoracic level. Pain travels from the heart to other body parts by triggering neural reflexes that activate the autonomic nervous system.

Angina can trigger excessive norepinephrine release, which causes platelet aggregation and thromboxane A release. Because metabolism becomes anaerobic, adenosine triphosphate production drops, allowing sodium to accumulate inside cells and potassium to collect outside. This chain of events impedes the heart's sequence of depolarization and repolarization, necessary for normal contraction.

Coronary Artery Disease/Angina

Continued on page 44

Assessing angina: Asking the right questions

- Where's the discomfort? Point to it.
- How would you describe the discomfort?
- How did it start? What brings it on? What relieves it?
- Does the discomfort seem to move? Where?
- Have you had the same discomfort before? How long did it last?
- Do you have any other symptoms of discomfort?

Questions that help distinguish angina from noncardiac pain

- Does the discomfort change or worsen when you shift position? (Angina isn't affected by body position changes.)
- Does respiration make the discomfort better or worse? (Angina isn't aggravated by respiration.)
- Can you point to the discomfort with one finger? (Angina tends to be diffuse, not sharply localized.)
- Does the discomfort seem deep or close to the surface? (Angina seems deep.)
- Does the discomfort seem intense, sharp, dull, or knifelike? (Angina's typically described as a dull ache, seldom sharp or stabbing.)

athy, mitral valve disease, and systemic lupus erythematosus may lead to angina. Signs and symptoms may also result from fever, anemia, tachydysrhythmias, hypotension, thyrotoxicosis, and polycythemia. About 5% to 10% of angina patients have coronary artery spasm, which can affect normal or occluded arteries.

Tracing angina's origins. The heart gets oxygen-rich blood from the coronary arteries. At rest, the heart takes about 75% of the circulatory system's oxygen, leaving 25% for the other organs. This leaves the heart little oxygen reserve when it's under stress, forcing it to rely on increased coronary blood flow to meet these extra needs. But atherosclerosis decreases blood flow. Increasing aortic pressure (to overcome vascular resistance created by the obstruction) may help, but not enough to meet myocardial oxygen demands during stress. The heart tries to compensate by dilating collateral vessels.

Heart rate, ventricular wall tension, and the heart's contractile state determine myocardial oxygen demand. During an angina attack, heart rate quickens, systemic blood pressure rises, and left ventricular end-diastolic pressure increases. But coronary artery lesions cause segmental myocardial dysfunction, even with increased collateral circulation. That dysfunction corrects itself once myocardial oxygen demands drop and coronary blood flow increases.

Assessment

A careful history of an angina pectoris patient can usually tell you more than a physical examination. *Remember, if your patient complains of chest pain, assume he's had an MI until proven otherwise.*

The questions you ask when taking the history can prove crucial. Find out what type of chest pain he's experiencing, note its location and duration, what preceded it, and what relieved it.

- *Type of pain.* The patient will probably describe angina pain as pressure, tightness, or a crushing, squeezing, or burning sensation. Angina pain's rarely called knifelike, sharp, or shooting. The patient may clench his fist against his chest while describing the pain.
- *Location.* Most patients feel angina pain in the substernal area. It may also radiate to the arms, neck, jaw, or back. (More localized pain's usually not cardiac-related.)
- *Duration.* Angina pain usually continues steadily, with only gradual intensity changes. It rarely fluctuates and may last 15 minutes or less. The longer the duration, the greater the chance of irreversible ischemia.
- *Precipitating events.* Typical angina triggers include any activity that places a greater-than-normal work load on the heart. Physical or emotional stress, exposure to extreme temperature changes, and eating a large meal can trigger pain.
- *Pain relief.* If the pain subsides within about 5 minutes of resting or taking nitroglycerin, suspect angina.

Be sure to observe your patient when taking his history. Does he clench his fist or lay his hand across his chest when he's in pain?

Continued on page 44

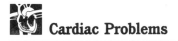
Coronary Artery Disease/Angina

Ischemia pain referral sites

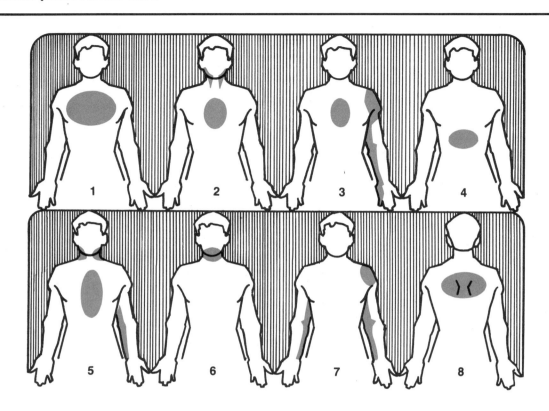

1. Upper chest

2. Beneath sternum, radiating to neck and jaw

3. Beneath sternum, radiating down left arm

4. Epigastric

5. Epigastric, radiating to neck, jaw, and arms

6. Neck and jaw

7. Left shoulder, inner aspect of both arms

8. Intrascapular

Angina—*continued*

Does he look pale? Is he diaphoretic? Does he have difficulty breathing? These signs and symptoms usually subside as the pain stops. Also identify any CAD risk factors in your patient's history.

Diagnostic studies. To help diagnose angina, the doctor may order a 12-lead EKG, chest X-ray, echocardiogram, radionuclide scans, and cardiac catheterization with coronary angiography. He may also order blood tests such as complete blood count, serum cholesterol, and lipid profile. Cardiac isoenzyme tests, if ordered, usually show normal values. (See the next few pages for details on angina diagnosis. Also read Chapter 2 for more information about cardiac diagnostic tests.)

Planning

Because all angina types stem from an imbalance of myocardial oxygen demand and supply, consider increasing supply or decreasing demand your priority. *Important:* Suspect an MI in an angina patient—especially if the angina's unstable—until proven otherwise.

Base your care plan on relieving pain and protecting the myocardium. After the patient's condition stablilizes, educate him and his

Coronary Artery Disease/Angina

A diagnostic option: Rapid atrial pacing

Some doctors use rapid atrial pacing instead of an exercise EKG test to diagnose angina because it allows them to investigate left ventricular function without the accompanying changes in cardiac output, afterload, and circulating catecholamines.

This test involves threading one end of a pacing wire into the patient's right atrium and attaching the other end to a pulse generator. Pacing usually starts at 100 beats per minute and increases by 20 beats every 2 minutes, up to a maximum of 160 beats.

EKGs taken after each 2-minute increase can detect ST segment depression and other ischemia indications. Pacing stops if the patient has chest pain or if ST depression appears. A positive test shows an ST depression of 1 mm, 0.08 seconds after the J point (where the QRS complex ends and the ST segment begins).

family about the disease, including its treatment and prevention. Also help him modify his life-style to reduce risk factors.

Nursing diagnoses. Possible nursing diagnoses for the angina pectoris patient may include:
- comfort, alteration in (chest pain); related to myocardial ischemia
- cardiac output, alteration in (decreased); related to atherosclerosis or coronary artery spasm
- knowledge deficit; related to disease and/or treatment
- coping, ineffective individual (or family); related to diagnosis
- family dynamics, alteration in; related to diagnosis
- noncompliance of treatment; related to inadequate health teaching
- anxiety, potential for; related to angina symptoms and underlying disease
- tissue perfusion, alteration in (cardiopulmonary); related to decreased cardiac output.

Below, you'll find a sample nursing care plan for the patient with stable angina. The plan lists expected outcomes, nursing interventions, and discharge planning that may be relevant to your patient. Remember to tailor each care plan to the needs of the patient and his family or support persons.

Continued on page 46

Sample nursing care plan—angina pectoris (stable)

Nursing diagnosis	Expected outcomes
Comfort, alteration in, (chest pain); related to myocardial ischemia.	The patient will: • Maintain an adequate comfort level. • Express relief and/or absence of pain. • Show knowledge of the rationale for antianginal medication. • Show knowledge of activities that reduce oxygen consumption.

Nursing interventions	Discharge planning
• Assess for verbal and nonverbal signs and symptoms of chest pain and associated signs and symptoms. • Monitor vital signs and EKG for evidence of changes before or during chest pain. • Instruct the patient to notify the nurse if chest pain occurs. • Provide emotional support during chest pain episodes. • Provide information about and maintain activities that reduce oxygen consumption. • After giving pain medication, check vital signs for indications of hypotension, and observe for pain relief and adverse medication effects. • Help patient recognize precipitating events and control angina attacks.	• Teach patient about controllable risk factors, such as smoking, hypertension, serum cholesterol levels, diabetes, obesity, lack of exercise, and stress. • Teach patient about his medications. • Teach patient specific activities and precautions to carry out at home, such as avoiding fatigue, sudden outbursts of emotions or activity, sports requiring much running or raising arms above the head, heavy lifting, extreme temperature changes, constipation, and excessive alcohol intake. • Teach patient about resumption of sexual activities and appropriate precautions, such as taking antianginal medication before sex and avoiding sex for at least 2 hours after meals.

Coronary Artery Disease/Angina

Angina—*continued*

Intervention
Management of angina pectoris may include:
- correcting CAD risk factors
- life-style changes
- medications
- PTCA or CABG.

Correcting risk factors. Help your patient change his habits to reduce his CAD risk. If he smokes, explain how smoking damages his cardiovascular system. If he's hypertensive, make sure he understands the importance of blood pressure monitoring and control. Encourage a diabetic patient to comply with dietary changes and oral hypoglycemic or insulin therapy to help control his serum glucose level. If the patient's obese or has high serum lipid levels, stress the need to limit intake of foods high in fat and carbohydrates.

An angina patient can benefit from prescribed and closely monitored exercises. Tell him to keep his activity level below that which triggers an angina attack and to avoid isometric exercise, which greatly increases myocardial oxygen demand.

Life-style changes. These include nonpharmacologic methods, for example, avoidance of stress, fatigue, extreme temperatures, large meals, and situations that provoke angina.

Your patient can probably enjoy normal sexual relations as long as he takes medication appropriately and engages in sex only when rested and free of emotional stress. Taking nitroglycerin before sex may help prevent pain.

Help your patient ward off angina attacks by giving support and encouragement as he begins the difficult task of changing a lifetime of habits. Make a special effort to educate his family members and close friends—your patient's support structure after he leaves the hospital.

Medications. Teach the angina patient how to use medications that may reduce pain duration and intensity during an attack; decrease the frequency of attacks; or prevent or delay the onset of MI. Most angina patients use nitrates, which relax smooth muscles. This dilates vessels, which decreases vascular resistance and lowers blood pressure, thus reducing the heart's work load. The doctor may order nitroglycerin, a fast-acting nitrate, and isosorbide, a long-acting nitrate. If nitroglycerin doesn't relieve acute pain, the doctor may order morphine sulfate. Morphine changes the patient's perception of pain, reduces anxiety and fear, induces sleep, causes venous pooling, and reduces myocardial oxygen demands.

The doctor may also order beta blockers, with or without nitrates, to decrease myocardial oxygen demand. These drugs block the myocardial response to sympathetic stimulation, decreasing oxygen demand and relieving anginal pain. Monitor the patient carefully for bradycardia, hypotension, and signs of congestive heart failure while he's receiving these drugs.

Nursing tip
If your patient has angina at night, tilt his bed 10° so that his feet point downhill. This lowers venous and arterial pressure around the heart and reduces the amount of blood returning to the heart.

Understanding nitrate action

Well known for their vasodilatory effects, nitrates relieve angina primarily through preload reduction. (Preload refers to the amount of ventricular stretch, caused by blood volume, in the left ventricle at the end of diastole.)

Nitrates reduce preload by dilating the venous system, reducing the amount of blood returned to the heart. Because the ventricle contains less blood, wall tension decreases and ventricular contraction requires less exertion. This reduces myocardial oxygen needs.

Nitrates also boost collateral blood flow, improving circulation to ischemic areas.

Coronary Artery Disease/Angina

Calcium channel blockers, the newest antianginal agents, block the flow of calcium ions across myocardial cell membranes, thus dilating coronary arteries, collateral vessels, and peripheral arteries and decreasing the heart's contractile force and work load. The FDA has approved three calcium channel blockers—verapamil, nifedipine, and diltiazem—for angina pectoris.

PTCA and CABG. The angina patient may require PTCA or CABG, discussed earlier in this chapter.

Evaluation

Base your evaluation of the angina patient on his expected patient outcomes, as listed on your nursing care plan. To determine whether your patient's improved, ask yourself these questions:
• Can he maintain an adequate comfort level?
• Does he know why and how to take his medication and how to identify any adverse effects?
• Does he know which activities will help reduce his heart's oxygen consumption?
• Does he know how to avoid the conditions that trigger his chest pain?

These questions, based on the care plan on page 45, may not apply to your patient. Remember to tailor your plan to the needs of your patient and his family.

Angina types

Angina usually takes one of three main forms:
Stable (chronic) angina pain occurs at a predictable level of physical or emotional stress, builds gradually, and quickly reaches maximum intensity. Pain generally lasts only a few minutes. Strenuous activity, cold weather, or heightened emotional stress may trigger stable angina. Rest or nitroglycerin tablets typically relieve it.

The patient may describe stable angina as a strangling sensation accompanied by anxiety, a crushing, viselike pain, or a tightness, heaviness, or squeezing sensation in the chest. Sometimes stable angina causes only a mild sensation of pressure.

The patient may have trouble pinpointing the discomfort site, but he'll probably indicate the substernal area, with radiation to the left arm, jaw, and neck and possibly to the right arm and back. He may also have shortness of breath, diaphoresis, faintness, anxiety, and nausea. Stable angina most frequently arises from coronary artery atherosclerosis.

Diagnosis of stable angina combines the patient's signs and symptoms with a detailed history, physical examination, and diagnostic testing. Although the EKG remains the most common test for ischemic heart disease, a resting EKG of a stable angina patient usually won't yield definitive proof. An exercise stress test may show the characteristic ST segment depression of ischemic heart disease. Studies show that a downsloping ST segment or horizontal ST segment depression specifically indicates CAD and appears frequently in patients with double- and triple-vessel disease, especially at low exercise levels.

Continued on page 48

Coronary Artery Disease/Angina

Transdermal nitroglycerin patches

The transdermal nitroglycerin patch changed long-term treatment of angina pectoris when it came on the scene a few years ago. Since then, some things about the patch have changed. Here's an update.

Patches now come in three brands—Nitrodisc, Nitro-Dur, and Transderm-Nitro—each releasing a constant stream of nitroglycerin into the bloodstream over a 24-hour period.

Therapy usually begins with a dose of 5 mg/24 hours. The dose increases gradually until the drug controls angina. The ideal dose reduces resting blood pressure as much as possible without producing orthostatic hypotension.

The patient may use one or more patches to deliver his daily dose. He may even mix and match different brands thanks to recent label standardization. All three brands now tell how much nitroglycerin they release over 24 hours. So if a patient's dose is 7.5 mg/24 hours, he can use a 5 mg/24 hours patch from one company and a 2.5 mg/24 hours patch from another.

Tell the patient to apply the patch to his chest, upper leg, back, or upper arm at the same time each day, using a different site each day. Warn him not to apply it to his lower leg or arm because these areas don't permit adequate drug absorption. To make sure the patch adheres properly, tell him to place it on a clean, dry, hairless site, avoiding skin that's scarred, callused, or irritated. Warn him not to cut the patch to reduce the dose. If the patch falls off, he should apply a new one.

Remind your patient that the patches help prevent angina, but won't treat acute attacks. To relieve an attack, he should carry sublingual nitroglycerin with him.

Transdermal nitroglycerin patches cause few adverse effects—most commonly, headache.

Nursing tip

To prevent complications during cardioversion or defibrillation, remove your patient's transdermal nitroglycerin patch before the procedures. The patch's backing, made from aluminum or an aluminized plastic, can conduct electricity, causing an explosion during defibrillation or cardioversion. More important, the patch could prevent successful cardioversion.

Angina types—*continued*

Holter monitoring also helps evaluate ischemia. Many stable angina patients show ST segment depression with certain activities even when they don't have chest pain. Stress thallium scans can distinguish between ischemic and infarcted heart tissue and aid prognosis.

Exercise radionuclide angiography and coronary angiography also help diagnose stable angina. Cardiac enzyme tests can help the doctor differentiate between angina and acute MI; levels for angina patients fall within normal range.

Treatment for stable angina focuses on balancing oxygen delivery with demand. In a stepped drug therapy, patients initially receive nitrates. Next, the doctor adds a beta blocker and, finally, calcium channel blockers. When caring for a stable angina patient, help him reduce or eliminate CAD risk factors.

Unstable angina, more severe than stable angina, frequently precedes an MI. Also called preinfarction angina, crescendo angina, acute coronary insufficiency, intermediate coronary syndrome, or impending MI, unstable angina takes an unpredictable course.

An imbalance between myocardial oxygen demand and supply, coronary artery spasm, stress-related catecholamine release, and platelet aggregation may contribute to this angina type.

One or more of these features characterize unstable angina:
• angina pectoris of new onset, brought on by minimal exertion
• increasingly severe, prolonged, or frequent angina in a pattern of relatively stable, exertion-related angina
• angina both at rest and during minimal exercise.

Unlike stable angina, unstable angina doesn't require such triggers as anemia, infection, thyrotoxicosis, or cardiac dysrhythmias. The pain resembles stable angina pain, although it's usually more intense, may last up to 30 minutes, and may arouse the patient from sleep.

The discomfort may occur with shortness of breath, nausea and/or vomiting, and diaphoresis and may radiate into previously uninvolved areas. Nitroglycerin may give only partial relief; some patients require narcotics.

The EKG usually diagnoses unstable angina, showing transient changes in the ST segment—either elevation or depression. Even if the EKG doesn't show these changes, the doctor can make a diagnosis based on the patient's history and clinical condition. He may also order the diagnostic tests described for stable angina.

To manage the unstable angina patient, promote coronary perfusion, relieve pain, and minimize pain recurrence. The patient will probably stay in the coronary care unit for close observation. The doctor will prescribe bed rest and oxygen to promote coronary perfusion. As ordered, give nitrates, such as nitroglycerin I.V., and narcotics, such as morphine, to relieve pain. The patient may also require sedation.

Coronary Artery Disease/Angina

The ergonovine test

To diagnose coronary artery spasm, the doctor may perform the highly sensitive ergonovine test. An ergot alkaloid, ergonovine causes direct vascular smooth muscle constriction, inducing coronary artery spasm in variant angina patients. I.V. doses ranging from 0.05 to 0.40 mg can trigger spasm. Vessels most prone to spontaneous spasm show the greatest sensitivity to the drug.

To minimize the risk of myocardial infarction, the doctor will use the ergonovine test only on a patient with normal or nearly normal coronary arteries. He'll give ergonovine in gradually increasing doses.

The test usually takes place in the cardiac catheterization laboratory, where personnel can diagnose the spasm angiographically and administer intracoronary nitroglycerin if needed to stop the spasm. Resuscitative equipment and medication must be on hand.

The test can also take place in the coronary care unit, although perhaps not as safely. Chest pain and ST-segment depression on EKG indicate a positive test.

To prevent further pain, the doctor may prescribe a regimen of nitrates, beta blockers, and/or calcium channel blockers—effective in about 75% of patients. The remaining patients need more aggressive intervention such as CABG, PTCA, or use of an intraaortic balloon pump.

Variant angina, which occurs at rest, presumably stems from coronary artery spasm. Also called Prinzmetal's angina, this syndrome usually doesn't result from exertion or stress and may arise without coronary atherosclerosis. Variant angina patients frequently lack CAD risk factors, although some smoke heavily. Attacks commonly come at the same time every day—frequently between midnight and 8 a.m.

Signs and symptoms of variant angina resemble those of unstable angina. The patient may complain of sudden substernal chest pain, ranging from a feeling of heaviness to a crushing discomfort. He may also experience shortness of breath, nausea and vomiting, and diaphoresis. Many variant angina patients have dysrhythmias and conduction abnormalities. Occasionally, a patient has both variant and stable exertional angina. Nitroglycerin generally gives prompt relief.

Acute MI may accompany variant angina. Roughly 15% of variant angina patients die suddenly.

To diagnose variant angina, the doctor will order an EKG, which typically shows a sudden, marked ST elevation during chest pain episodes that quickly disappears with pain relief. In a patient with suspected coronary spasm, coronary angiography may help identify angina's cause by reproducing the spasm. Ergonovine maleate, methacholine, or histamine induce coronary artery spasm in a variant angina patient. The doctor may also order the tests described for stable angina.

Care for the variant angina patient as you'd care for a stable angina patient. But keep in mind the treatment goal: to prevent coronary artery spasm. Administer nitrates and calcium channel blockers, as ordered. (But keep in mind that nitrates work in variant angina patients by directly dilating coronary arteries rather than reducing myocardial oxygen demands.) Beta-adrenergic blockers can constrict coronary vessels, so the doctor probably won't order them. Calcium channel blockers help prevent coronary artery spasm by dilating these vessels and inhibiting contraction. (*Note:* Variant angina patients typically don't need surgery because they usually don't have CAD.)

Myocardial Infarction: When Cells Die

Myocardial infarction (MI) tops the list of leading causes of death in the U.S. About half of MI patients die within an hour of MI onset. Although those who receive immediate care stand a greater survival chance, 10% to 15% will die in the hospital or within the next year.

What brings on MI? It usually begins with atherosclerosis—the main cause of coronary artery disease (CAD). But an MI can arise from *any* condition in which myocardial oxygen supply can't keep pace with demand; for instance, severe coronary artery spasm or coronary artery thrombosis. Starved of oxygen, the myocardium suffers progressive ischemia, leading to injury and, finally, to infarction.

Other MI causes include surgery or trauma with acute blood loss and, less commonly, coronary artery embolism, dissecting aortic aneurysm, polyarteritis nodosa, neoplasm, or radiation therapy.

Atherosclerosis-induced MI comes about in this way: Plaques (atherosclerotic lesions) increasingly narrow the coronary artery, eventually occluding blood flow. Blood cells rushing past the roughened, calcified plaques cause the plaques to break apart. In response, platelets aggregate, stimulating release of the prostaglandin throm-

Sharon and John VanRiper, who wrote this chapter, work at the University of Michigan Medical Center in Ann Arbor. Sharon, who received her MS degree from the University, is assistant head nurse. John, who earned his BSN degree from Wayne State University in Detroit, is a surgical intensive care nurse.

Some MI causes in patients without atherosclerosis

Coronary artery disease (other than atherosclerosis):
• arteritis
• trauma to coronary arteries
• coronary mural thickening with metabolic diseases or intimal proliferative disease
• luminal narrowing by other mechanisms, such as spasm of coronary arteries (Prinzmetal's angina), spasm after nitroglycerin withdrawal, aortic dissection, and coronary artery dissection.

Coronary artery emboli:
• infective endocarditis
• cardiac myxoma
• cardiopulmonary bypass surgery and coronary arteriography.

Congenital coronary artery anomalies

Myocardial oxygen demand-supply imbalance:
• aortic stenosis
• aortic insufficiency
• carbon monoxide poisoning
• thyrotoxicosis
• prolonged hypotension.

Hematologic causes:
• polycythemia vera
• thrombocytosis
• disseminated intravascular coagulation
• hypercoagulability
• thrombosis
• thrombocytopenic purpura.

Miscellaneous causes:
• myocardial contusion
• MI with normal coronary arteries.

The ravages of MI

Myocardial tissue destruction, caused by a halt in myocardial blood supply, significantly alters cardiodynamics, decreasing cardiac output. Compensatory mechanisms intensify oxygen demand, destroying more myocardial tissue. The patient's prognosis depends on the extent of tissue involved, its remaining contractility, and the effectiveness of its inflammatory response. Here's how an MI develops:

Injury to the coronary artery's intimal lining increases endothelial cell membrane permeability. The arterial lumen narrows as platelets, white blood cells, fibrin, and lipids adhere to the injury site.

Meantime, collateral circulation helps maintain myocardial perfusion distal to the obstruction.

However, stress creates a greater myocardial oxygen demand than collaterals can supply. Myocardial metabolism, normally aerobic, shifts to anaerobic producing lactic acid, which stimulates pain nerve endings.

Oxygen deficit causes myocardial cell death, which leads to decreased contractility, stroke volume, and blood pressure. Hypotension stimulates baroreceptors, triggering release of epinephrine and neuroepinephrine. These catecholamines boost the heart rate and peripheral vasoconstriction, further intensifying myocardial oxygen demand.

Damaged cell membranes in the infarcted area spill their contents into the systemic vascular circulation.

Myocardial Infarction

Other MI sites

Not all MIs occur in the left ventricle. Other possible sites include the right ventricle and the atria. Right ventricular MI can arise independently. However, it's more likely to develop with an inferior or posterior left ventricular MI, because the right coronary artery and its posterior descending branch perfuse these areas.

Suspect right ventricular MI if your patient has signs and symptoms of unexplained right heart failure, such as neck vein distention, increased right atrial pressure, or right ventricular S_3 or S_4. Hemodynamic pressures and radionuclide imaging may aid diagnosis. The 12-lead EKG rarely diagnoses right ventricular infarction because its leads orient to the left ventricle.

As your first priority in caring for a patient with right ventricular MI, administer fluids, as ordered, to maintain or improve left ventricular filling. This optimizes cardiac output. Avoid giving diuretics because they reduce right ventricular filling pressures by decreasing circulating blood volume.

Atrial MI may occur with left ventricular MI or obstructive disease of the sinus node artery. Frequently accompanied by atrial dysrhythmias, an atrial MI usually occurs on the right side, in the atrial appendages. An atrial MI can result in atrial wall rupture.

EKG evidence of an atrial MI includes: depressed or elevated PR intervals, altered P-wave configurations, and ectopic atrial rhythms such as atrial fibrillation, atrial flutter, or wandering pacemaker.

Treatment of both right ventricular and atrial MI centers on relieving symptoms and preventing complications.

Pinpointing MI location and size

An MI's location and size depend on one or more of the following:
• the location and severity of atherosclerosis
• the presence, site, and severity of coronary artery spasm
• the size of the vascular bed perfused by the narrowed vessel
• the extent of collateral circulation
• the oxygen demands of poorly perfused myocardium.

boxane A. This potent vasoconstrictor promotes formation of a thrombus, which may then circulate in the coronary arteries until reaching a part of the vessel too narrow to pass through. The thrombus lodges there, completely occluding the artery. Cells dependent on the occluded vessel for oxygen then become ischemic. If emergency intervention or collateral blood supply can't restore circulation to the involved tissue within 4 hours, cell injury progresses to cell death, signaling infarction.

Most MIs involve the left ventricle because this chamber has a thicker wall, larger perfusion area and vessel supply, and greater work load.

MI triggers the release of catecholamines, bringing on various changes. Mechanical changes including vasoconstriction and increased contractility can elevate blood pressure and increase cardiac output and myocardial oxygen use. Electrophysiologic changes include decreased conduction velocity and increased heart rate. Metabolic changes include increased serum glucose and free fatty acid (FFA) levels. Anxiety, a feeling of loss of control, and the fear of death can enhance the other effects.

Continued on page 52

Left ventricle MIs

MIs occur in two main types—transmural and subendocardial (nontransmural). Usually indicated by its location in the left ventricle (anterior, inferior, posterior, or lateral wall), transmural MI involves the full myocardial thickness. Anterior wall MI poses the gravest risk, as it usually affects a larger region and frequently triggers dysrhythmias. Subendocardial MI arises in the superficial region of the ventricle's inner lining. Other MI types include endocardial, subepicardial, and intramural.

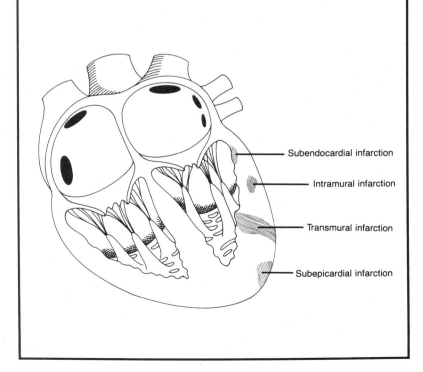

Subendocardial infarction

Intramural infarction

Transmural infarction

Subepicardial infarction

Myocardial Infarction

Silent ischemia

Myocardial ischemia doesn't always make its presence known. Studies show that many MI patients lack indications of extensive coronary artery obstruction. Evidence of ischemia may appear only when a routine EKG reveals an old infarction or when death occurs.

Why does one patient lack symptoms while another experiences warning signs? The patient with silent ischemia may have a higher pain threshold or an autonomic neuropathy related to diabetes. Or he may have a smaller ischemic area. Others with silent ischemia deny their symptoms.

Although no large-scale studies have investigated the prognosis for patients with silent ischemia, some data suggest that they stand a better survival chance than those with known arterial obstruction.

Emergency MI intervention

If you suspect your patient's had an MI, act quickly by taking the following steps:
• Notify the doctor immediately.
• Administer oxygen by mask or nasal cannula, as ordered.
• Establish an I.V. line, as ordered.
• Run a 12-lead EKG.
• Be prepared to administer nitroglycerin and/or an analgesic such as morphine, as ordered.
• Gather emergency equipment.
• Remain calm and reassure the patient.

Besides an EKG, the doctor may also order cardiac enzyme, arterial blood gas (ABG), complete blood count (CBC), and serum electrolyte tests to determine the location and extent of MI damage.

Continued

Pathologic changes. Myocardial changes don't appear until about 6 hours after an MI. The affected area swells slightly and appears pale and bluish. About 18 to 36 hours later, the myocardium turns tan or reddish purple. An epicardial exudate may develop after transmural MI. Two days later, the MI site turns gray and fine yellow lines appear at the damaged site's periphery. In the next few days, the gray area broadens, eventually to the entire MI area.

Mononuclear cells phagocytize the necrotic tissue 8 to 10 days after MI, reducing cardiac wall thickness in the infarct area. A reddish purple band of granulated tissue pervades the region. In 3 to 4 weeks, the MI area takes on a gelatinous, gray look and develops scar tissue. The endocardium beneath the infarct thickens, turning gray and opaque.

Collateral circulation usually increases in the first few weeks after MI. Although collaterals may help limit infarct size, they can't always meet a stressed heart's needs and may not prevent myocardial necrosis.

Assessment

A patient with a suspected MI will usually complain of chest pain. Find out the following information when taking his history.
• *Type of pain.* MI usually causes a heavy-pressure, crushing, or squeezing pain unaffected by changes in body position or respiration. However, many MI patients have only mild or vague discomfort resembling indigestion.
• *Location.* Suspect an MI if the patient complains of substernal pain or pain radiating to the arm (particularly the left arm), neck, jaw, or back.
• *Duration.* Sudden onset of pain that's continuous and prolonged suggests MI.
• *Precipitating events.* Stress, anxiety, exertion, temperature changes, and overeating typically bring on MI pain.
• *Relieving factors.* Rest and nitroglycerin usually don't relieve MI pain.

If you suspect an MI, intervene quickly by taking the nursing actions described in *Emergency MI intervention.*

Physical examination. As you give emergency care, also assess the patient for these signs and symptoms of an MI and possible complications:

General appearance. An MI patient usually appears anxious, restless, or apprehensive. He may clench his chest or experience shortness of breath, nausea, or vomiting. His skin may turn gray and ashen. Check for marked jugular vein distention—a sign of right ventricular infarction or congestive heart failure.

Vital signs. The MI patient's pulse may be rapid, irregular, or slow. Check the carotid pulse. If it's hard to detect, suspect reduced stroke volume. Next, check the patient's blood pressure. After MI, blood pressure may drop from decreased cardiac output, vagal tone, or pain. Also expect an increased respiratory rate, resulting from pain and anxiety. A fever may appear in the first 24 to 48 hours after MI from the tissue necrosis or inflammation of acute pericarditis.

Chest palpation. Expect a palpable precordial pulse in an MI patient.

Auscultation. If your patient's had an MI, you may hear only muffled heart sounds until the myocardium heals. If you detect a third heart

Myocardial Infarction

sound (S₃), suspect extensive ventricular dysfunction, decreased compliance, or ventricular dilatation. A fourth heart sound (S₄) reflects reduced left ventricular compliance. Crackles in the lung bases may indicate left ventricular failure.

Diagnostic studies. If your patient's history or physical examination suggests MI, observe him closely throughout diagnostic testing. The doctor will order an electrocardiogram (EKG), cardiac enzyme analysis, other blood tests, and radionuclide studies to confirm MI.

EKG. Serial EKG tracings yield the best evidence of MI. A transmural MI produces pathologic Q waves, ST-segment changes, and T-wave changes. (See chart below for more information.) Normally, MI progresses through the following EKG phases in the leads showing the MI:

Continued on page 54

Telltale EKG findings: The three I's of an MI

Ischemia, injury, and infarction (the three I's of an MI) produce characteristic EKG changes, as explained below:

• *Ischemia* temporarily interrupts blood supply to myocardial tissue but generally doesn't cause cell death.

EKG changes: T-wave inversion, resulting from altered tissue repolarization. (See waveform at top right.)

• *Injury* results from prolonged blood supply interruption, causing further cell injury.

EKG changes: elevated ST segment, resulting from altered depolarization. Consider an elevation greater than 1 mm significant. (See middle waveform.)

• *Infarction* ensues from complete lack of blood reaching the cell. This causes myocardial cell death (necrosis).

EKG changes: pathologic Q wave (or QS), resulting from abnormal depolarization or from scar tissue that can't depolarize. Look for Q-wave duration of 0.04 seconds or more or an amplitude measuring at least a third of the QRS complex.

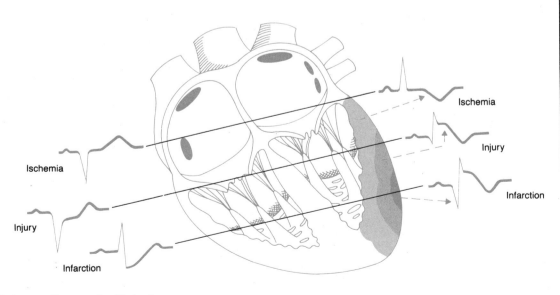

Changes on the opposite side (reciprocal changes)

Changes on the damaged side

Myocardial Infarction

Identifying MI damage site

Use this chart to identify MI damage location. But remember, myocardial damage may spread to other areas. (*Note:* EKG changes occurring in the acute phase include pathologic Q wave, ST-segment elevation, and T-wave inversion.)

Wall affected	Leads	Possible EKG changes	Possible coronary artery involved	Possible reciprocal changes
Inferior (diaphragmatic)	II, III, aVF	Q, ST, T	RCA	I, aVL
Lateral	I, aVL, V_5, V_6	Q, ST, T	Circumflex, branch of LAD	V_1, V_3
Anterior	V_1, V_2, V_3, V_4, I, aVL	Q, ST, T, loss of R-wave progression	LCA	II, III, aVF
Posterior	V_1, V_2	R greater than S, ST depression, elevated T wave (mirror change)	RCA, circumflex	
Apical	V_3, V_4, V_5, V_6	Q, ST, T, loss of R-wave progression	LAD, RCA	
Anterolateral	I, aVL, V_4, V_5, V_6	Q, ST, T	LAD, circumflex	II, III, aVF
Anteroseptal	V_1, V_2, V_3	Q, ST, T, loss of septal R wave in V_1	LAD	
Subendocardial	Any of the above	ST, T for more than 3 days with enzyme changes		

Continued

• hyperacute phase (begins a few hours after MI): ST-segment elevation and upright T waves
• fully evolved phase (starts hours after MI onset): deep T-wave inversion and pathologic Q waves
• resolution phase (appears within a few weeks after MI): normal T waves
• stabilized chronic phase (follows the resolution phase): permanent pathologic Q waves revealing an old infarction.

An EKG can also show reciprocal changes recorded from leads opposite the damaged region.

A subendocardial MI will produce persistent ST-segment depression or T-wave inversion, or both. Q waves may not appear. Factors that may limit an EKG's diagnostic value for MI extent and location include conduction defects, previous MIs, acute pericarditis, electrolyte imbalances, and cardioactive drug use.

Cardiac enzyme analysis. About 30 to 60 minutes after irreversible injury to myocardial tissue, certain enzymes and their isoenzymes (molecularly distinct subtypes) spill into the plasma. Findings indicating MI include elevated creatine phosphokinase (CPK or CK), lactic dehydrogenase (LDH), and serum glutamic-oxaloacetic transaminase levels (SGOT). Most doctors consider the pattern of enzyme levels when looking for evidence of MI.

Myocardial Infarction

About 6 to 8 hours after MI, CPK levels rise, peaking in about 24 hours. They usually return to normal 3 to 4 days after chest pain begins. (Normally, total CPK values range from 23 to 99 u/liter in men and 15 to 57 u/liter in women.)

Although CPK gives the most accurate indication of MI, levels may be high for other reasons, including skeletal muscle disease or trauma, acute alcohol intoxication, diabetes mellitus, vigorous exercise, convulsions, I.M. injections, pulmonary embolism, or central nervous system disorders.

CPK has three isoenzymes. CPK-MB concentrates mainly in the heart; CPK-BB in the brain; and CPK-MM in skeletal muscle. CPK-MB elevation gives the best enzymatic evidence of MI. It rises markedly 4 to 8 hours after MI onset, peaks at 18 to 24 hours, and may stay high for up to 72 hours. However, CPK-MB may also rise from myocarditis, CPR, and cardiac trauma (including trauma from catheterization and surgery). Normally, CPK-MB values range from undetectable to 7 IU/liter.

Because LDH exceeds the normal range 24 to 48 hours after MI and peaks in 3 to 6 days, LDH analysis can help confirm MI in a patient admitted to the hospital a day or more after chest pain onset. LDH values normally range from 48 to 115 IU/liter.

LDH has five organ-specific isoenzymes. LDH_1 and LDH_2 localize primarily in the heart, kidneys, and red blood cells; LDH_3 in the lungs; and LDH_4 and LDH_5 in the liver and skeletal muscles. Conditions other than MI that can elevate LDH include anemia, leukemia, liver disease, hepatic congestion, renal disease, neoplasms, pulmonary embolism, myocarditis, skeletal muscle disease, shock, and hemolysis.

Continued on page 56

Serum enzyme changes after transmural MI

The graph below shows how serum enzyme levels may change after a transmural MI.

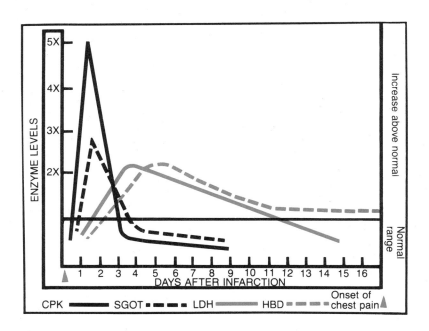

Myocardial Infarction

Continued

Normally, LDH$_2$ levels exceed LDH$_1$ levels. About 24 to 48 hours after MI, the pattern flips, with LDH$_1$ concentrations exceeding LDH$_2$ levels. Hemolytic anemia, hemolysis, renal infarction, hyperthyroidism, and stomach carcinoma can also flip the pattern.

To measure LDH$_2$ indirectly, the doctor may order a hydroxybutyric dehydrogenase (HBD) test. HBD, a property of the LDH enzyme, reflects LDH$_1$ activity. An HBD test may also substitute for an LDH enzyme fractionation study because it's cheaper and simpler to perform. However, HBD analysis can't distinguish between myocardial and liver damage as reliably. (Normal HBD values range from 114 to 290 u/ml. The ratio of LDH to HBD varies from 1:2 to 1.6:1.)

Found throughout the body, SGOT concentrates in the heart, liver, skeletal muscle, pancreas, kidneys, and lungs. Approximately 8 to 12 hours after the onset of chest pain, concentrations exceed the normal range, peak 18 to 36 hours later, and subside to normal within 3 to 4 days.

However, SGOT studies rank as the most insensitive and nonspecific of the cardiac enzyme tests, and many hospitals no longer perform them. Other disorders causing SGOT elevation include liver disease, skeletal muscle disease, I.M. injection, shock, pericarditis, and pulmonary embolism.

Other blood tests. MI may also alter findings for the following tests.

• *White blood cell (WBC) count.* Within approximately 2 hours after chest pain starts, WBC rises in response to tissue necrosis or increased secretion of adrenal glucocorticoids—or both. Generally, WBC peaks 2 to 4 days after MI and returns to normal a week later. Peak WBC usually ranges between 12×10^3 and 15×10^3 per mm^3. The percentage of polymorphonuclear leukocytes also rises, and the differential count shifts to band forms.

Comparing hot-spot and cold-spot imaging

The doctor may order either of these diagnostic tests if your patient has had an MI. Read what follows to learn how they differ.

Test	Purpose	Reliability	Disadvantages
99ᵐ technetium pyro-phosphate scan (hot-spot imaging)	• To detect irreversibly infarcted myocardium • To identify MI type, location, and size • To help confirm MI when: the EKG can't; the patient has a complete left bundle branch block; enzyme tests prove unreliable (for example, after cardiac surgery); pacemaker activity distorts MI changes.	Can detect MI 12 hours to 6 days later. Peak uptake occurs after about 36 hours. Scan's usually negative 7 to 10 days after MI.	Other pathologic conditions may appear as hot spots (for example, ventricular aneurysms, tumors, or other myocardial damage).
Thallium 201 scan (cold-spot imaging)	• To differentiate ischemic from normal or infarcted myocardium, especially when used in conjunction with exercise EKG • To evaluate blood flow through coronary arteries • To identify high-risk MI patients.	Can detect MI in its first few hours.	Results less specific and harder to interpret. Poorly perfused areas, electrodes, breast implants, and conditions such as sarcoidosis, cardiac contusion, and coronary spasm appear as cold spots. Test can't distinguish old from new MIs.

Myocardial Infarction

● *Erythrocyte sedimentation rate (ESR).* Approximately 4 or 5 days after MI, ESR may peak and may stay high for weeks. (Serum concentrations of copper and nickel parallel ESR elevations.)

● *Hematocrit.* This value may rise the first few days after MI from hemoconcentration.

Other findings. Myocardial cells release myoglobin into the blood a few hours after MI. Urinary myoglobin levels also rise markedly after MI. Hyperglycemia may also follow MI, along with decreased serum zinc, iron, and magnesium levels.

Radionuclide studies. Expect the doctor to order thallium scans, 99^m technetium pyrophosphate scans, or radionuclide ventriculography to evaluate MI effects. Radioimmunoassay (RIA), which detects cardiac myosin light chains (CM-LC), can also reveal early- and late-stage cardiac necrosis.

Cardiac catherization and angiography may also be ordered. (See Chapter 2 for more information on cardiac diagnostic tests.)

Planning
Before determining your nursing care plan, develop the nursing diagnosis by identifying the patient's problem—or potential problem—then relating the problem to its cause. Possible nursing diagnoses for an MI patient include the following:
● Cardiac output, alteration in (decreased); related to MI
● Comfort, alteration in (chest pain); related to myocardial hypoxia
● Tissue perfusion, alteration in (decreased); related to MI
● Anxiety; related to acute illness, fear of death, ICU environment
● Coping, ineffective family or individual; related to diagnosis
● Sexual dysfunction; related to fear of another MI
● Injury (cardiac dysrhythmias) potential for; related to myocardial ischemia.

The sample nursing care plan for an MI patient, below, shows expected outcomes, nursing interventions, and discharge planning for one of the nursing diagnoses listed above. You'll want to individualize each care plan, however, to fit the needs of the patient and his family.

Continued on page 58

Sample nursing care plan—Myocardial infarction

Nursing diagnosis	Expected outcomes
● Cardiac output, alteration in (decreased); related to myocardial infarction	The patient will: ● maintain adequate cardiac output and tissue perfusion without signs of heart failure ● maintain adequate blood pressure, heart rate, and urinary output.

Nursing interventions	Discharge planning
● Assess and record vital signs every hour, or as needed. ● Assess and record lung and heart sounds every hour, or as needed. Stay alert for crackles or extra heart sounds. ● Monitor dysrhythmias and record heart rhythm variations. ● Monitor for signs and symptoms of decreased cardiac output. ● Monitor and record fluid intake and output. ● Maintain urine output of at least 30 ml/hour.	● Assess the patient's ability to assume activities of daily living (ADL). Plan to gradually increase this level. ● Teach the patient about his prescribed medications and stress compliance with drug therapy. ● Instruct the patient to weigh himself daily and report changes of 3 lb. or more to the doctor. ● Tell the patient to report any difficulty in breathing or shortness of breath to the doctor. ● Teach the patient about the heart disease process.

Myocardial Infarction

Continued
Intervention
Initial treatment goals for the MI patient include:
- reducing pain
- preventing further myocardial damage
- maximizing tissue oxygenation
- minimizing myocardial oxygen consumption
- maintaining adequate cardiac output.

The doctor will place the patient on bed rest initially to reduce the heart's work load and give oxygen to increase tissue oxygenation.

Drugs. Expect the doctor to order narcotics, such as morphine sulfate or meperidine I.V.; nitrates; and beta blockers to decrease myocardial oxygen use and relieve pain and anxiety. Morphine's frequently preferred because it reduces oxygen demand, promotes vasodilation, and helps relieve anxiety. Nitroglycerin, given either I.V. or sublingually, in addition to reducing myocardial oxygen consumption and demand, may also lower the risk of ventricular dysrhythmias. (If possible, give drugs I.V. rather than I.M. to help prevent cardiac enzyme elevation and improve drug absorption.)

Beta blockers (such as propranolol and timolol) help protect ischemic myocardium from increased concentrations of circulating catecholamines and sympathetic nerve stimulation, which increase heart rate and contractility. Thus, they help reduce the risk of another MI.

Thrombolysis. If the patient's MI resulted from acute coronary thrombosis, the doctor may order thrombolytic drug therapy. When given promptly, thrombolytics can sometimes restore myocardial perfusion and prevent tissue death. Streptokinase, the most frequently used thrombolytic, activates plasmin—an enzyme that dissolves fibrin, the clot-forming substance. Urokinase, costlier but more potent than streptokinase, also promotes clot lysis.

Streptokinase, given I.V. or by intracoronary infusion, has proven most effective when administered within 4 hours after onset of chest pain. Intracoronary infusion requires cardiac catheterization for administration.

However, streptokinase can cause serious bleeding disorders. Check the patient's baseline coagulation studies before starting the drug. Avoid administering thrombolytics to a patient who's had surgery in the last 10 days, cerebrovascular accident, GI bleeding, or major trauma. Streptokinase also increases the risk of complications and death in a patient who later needs coronary artery bypass graft (CABG) surgery.

During and after thrombolytic therapy, observe your patient closely for signs and symptoms of bleeding: unexplained bruising, hemoptysis, hematuria, epistaxis, positive stool or gastric guaiac tests, or sudden changes in mood, mentation, or sensation.

Glucose-insulin-potassium infusion. This therapy, most effective within 6 hours of MI onset, reduces FFA concentrations and improves ventricular performance. The combined substances increase glucose transport into myocardial cells, providing a continuous fuel supply in anaerobic

Myocardial Infarction

New MI drugs

The investigational clot-dissolving drug known as tissue-type plasminogen activator (t-PA) may improve treatment of acute MI. Like intracoronary streptokinase, t-PA recanalizes coronary arteries. But because it can be administered I.V., it avoids the disadvantages of catheterization (required for intracoronary infusion). Most important, t-PA reduces the patient's bleeding risk. T-PA induces coronary thrombolysis without systemic fibrinogen inactivation in most patients.

Pro-UK, also under investigation, may help treat MI, deep-vein thrombosis, and pulmonary embolism. This fibrin-specific substance, a form of urokinase known also as kidney plasminogen activator, acts as a clot-lysing agent.

glycolysis. Glucose also aids aerobic metabolism. Potassium restores ionic gradients, thus reducing the risk of ventricular dysrhythmias, and may also lower plasma FFA levels by inhibiting intracellular lipolysis. Insulin improves myocardial perfusion and contractility.

Coronary artery bypass graft surgery or percutaneous transluminal coronary angioplasty (PTCA). These procedures help revascularize the myocardium and may prevent further MIs. (See Chapter 3 for more information on CABG and PTCA.)

Intraaortic balloon pumping (IABP). This procedure helps stabilize patients with cardiogenic shock or uncontrollable chest pain and those awaiting CABG surgery. (See Chapter 5 for more information on IABP.)

Continued on page 60

Coronary failure cycle in MI

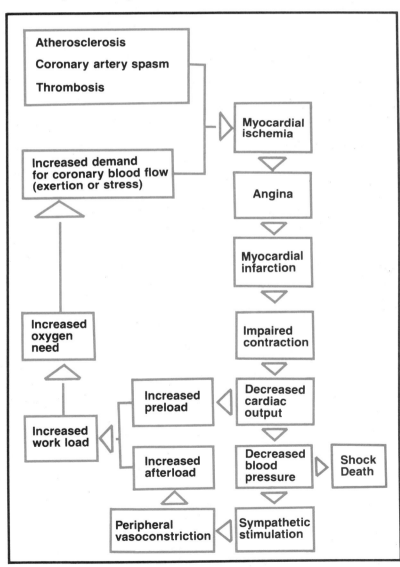

Myocardial Infarction

Continued

Complications

Dysrhythmias. These top the list of post-MI complications. Stay alert for:
- premature ventricular contractions (PVCs)
- ventricular tachycardia
- accelerated idioventricular rhythms, which may occur in the first 2 days after onset of chest pain, especially in a patient with an anterior or inferior MI
- ventricular fibrillation, also common after an anterior or inferior MI (but rare in subendocardial MI). *Note:* An MI patient with PVCs, ventricular tachycardia, or ventricular fibrillation stands a greatly increased risk of sudden death.

Premature atrial contractions and paroxysmal supraventricular tachycardia may also follow MI. A patient with an inferior wall MI may have first-degree AV block, Mobitz Type I second-degree AV block, or sinus bradycardia; anterior wall MI may lead to atrial fibrillation or Mobitz Type II second-degree AV block. Sinus tachycardia, commonly found with MI, increases oxygen consumption and reduces coronary perfusion.

Some patients with anterior or inferior MI develop complete AV heart block (CHB). CHB may develop gradually after an inferior wall MI. Anterior wall MI patients may develop CHB suddenly and face a greater risk of death.

Congestive heart failure (CHF). This disorder, which causes a third of all MI deaths, usually affects the left side because of the left ventricle's large muscle mass. CHF results from decreased contractility caused by myocardial tissue death. The amount of tissue death usually corresponds to the failure's severity.

Cardiogenic shock. This complication, which affects 10% to 20% of acute MI patients, results from depressed ventricular function, which results from loss of myocardial mass associated with necrosis of the left ventricle's muscle tissue.

Pericarditis. During the initial healing period, pericarditis may develop from pericardial irritation stemming from cellular debris and exudates in the infarct area. The condition may persist up to 3 months. Suspect pericarditis if your patient complains of atypical, long-lasting chest pain. He may also have a low-grade fever. EKG signs of pericarditis include persistent ST-segment elevation in leads facing the inflammation. Also check for pericardial friction rub.

Dressler's syndrome. Possibly arising from an autoimmune response or a virus, this disorder can occur 1 day to 3 months after MI. It may accompany pericarditis, pleurisy, or pneumonitis. Signs and symptoms include fever, chest pain, dyspnea, and EKG changes similar to those caused by pericarditis. Chest pain intensifies with thoracic movement and deep inspirations.

Thromboembolism. Mural thrombus formation in the left ventricle can lead to systemic embolism, while pulmonary embolism usually begins in deep leg veins. To reduce your patient's risk, encourage early ambulation.

Myocardial Infarction

Cost-cutting tip

To shorten the MI patient's stay in the intensive care unit, assess his status and anticipate complications immediately after he's been admitted.

Muscle dysfunction. The following muscle dysfunctions may occur after MI:
• Ventricular wall rupture, which leads to death from cardiac tamponade.
• Intraventricular septum rupture, generally occurring in the first week after MI. The rupture can cause congestive heart failure and shock.
• Ventricular aneurysm, possible weeks, months, or years after MI.
• Papillary muscle dysfunction, which may follow impaired blood flow to the large penetrating branches of the coronary arteries.
• Papillary muscle rupture, most frequent in the first week after MI. Rupture renders valve leaflets floppy and inefficient.

ICU psychosis. An MI patient may become confused and undergo personality changes from fear of death, loss of control, sleep deprivation, pain, or fear of monitors and other hospital equipment. Adverse effects of drugs, hypotension, impaired cerebral blood flow, and isolation from family can also cause ICU psychosis.

Cardiac cripple syndrome. Suspect this in a patient who resists resuming normal daily activities, from anxiety brought on by fear of death or disability.

Other complications. Hiccuping frequently accompanies inferior wall MIs. Nausea and vomiting can occur during an MI's acute phase. However, in later phases, analgesics and other cardiac drugs more frequently provoke these complications. Because retching can cause dysrhythmias, intervene promptly to relieve it.

Abdominal distention, constipation, and fecal impaction may result from lack of exercise, decreased dietary roughage, medication, or potassium depletion following diuresis. In a patient with a peptic ulcer, stress can trigger GI hemorrhaging.

Predicting the patient's recovery. An MI patient's prognosis depends on the amount of tissue necrosis, remaining left ventricular function (if the MI occurred in the left ventricle), and presence and severity of complications. A patient with an MI affecting large parts of the left ventricle will probably have decreased left ventricular contractility, which reduces cardiac output and may cause CHF and dysrhythmias. Studies show that patients with low ejection fractions (a measurement of left ventricular function) or complex ventricular dysrhythmias after MI risk sudden death within a year.

Risk factors such as uncontrolled hypertension, diabetes, hyperlipidemia, or smoking increase the chance of another MI. Make every effort to help the patient eliminate or reduce these factors.

Evaluation

Base your evaluation on the patient's expected outcome listed on your nursing care plan. To determine whether the patient's improved, ask yourself these questions:
• Can he maintain an adequate cardiac output?
• Does he have acceptable blood pressure, pulse, and urinary output?
• Does he have signs or symptoms of CHF?

The answers to these questions will help you evaluate your patient's care and determine his future needs. Keep in mind that these questions stem from the care plan shown on page 58. Your questions may differ.

Muscle Dysfunction: The Failing Pump

In this chapter, we'll review the most common types of cardiac muscle dysfunction—heart failure and cardiomyopathy.

Heart failure

Among the most common clinical problems you'll encounter, heart failure occurs when the heart can't pump enough blood to supply the needs of peripheral body tissues.

Heart failure may arise as a primary myocardial defect or as a consequence of other cardiac diseases such as valvular disease or cardiomyopathy. It can lead to distressing and potentially life-threatening symptoms in a patient of any age.

Understanding heart failure's origins and the pathophysiologic changes it brings about will prove essential to your care of a heart failure patient. You'll need to know how to differentiate right from left heart failure and high-output from low-output failure; gauge the patient's response to therapy; identify any acute changes; and predict the patient's expected outcome.

Heart failure's generally classified according to its primary location—in the right or left ventricle. One ventricle may fail independently of the other. But because the ventricles adjoin, blood travels in a constant circuit between the two. Thus, pump failure on one side frequently affects the other.

Because diseases such as coronary artery disease (CAD), hypertension, or valvular problems affect the left side more than the right, primary failure occurs more frequently on the left side. As blood backs up in the pulmonary vasculature and pressure builds, the right ventricle may also fail. (Congestive heart failure gets its name from the resulting pulmonary congestion.)

Connie Barden, a former cardiac clinical specialist at Mercy Hospital in Miami, wrote this chapter. She received her BSN from the University of North Carolina in Chapel Hill and her MSN from the University of Alabama in Birmingham.

Myofibril structure and function

Cardiac muscle cells consist of myofibrils—long, thin protein strands that contain the following:
• **Sarcomeres.** The muscle cell's functional units, these contain four proteins. *Myosin* has thick filaments running the length of the myofibril's A band. *Actin*, a thinner filament contained within the I band, extends from each end of the sarcomere. Actin overlaps and interconnects with myosin, forming dense areas in the A band. *Tropomyosin*, bound to actin, inhibits interaction between actin and myosin, causing muscle cell relaxation. *Troponin*, a globular protein, acts with tropomyosin to inhibit actin-myosin interaction.

• **Mitochondria.** These abundant cytoplasmic organelles produce energy in the form of adenosine triphosphate (ATP).

• **Sarcoplasmic reticulum.** This extensive intracellular network regulates calcium concentrations in the cell and plays a key role in muscle excitation.

• **T tubules.** These form a pathway for action potentials. Electrical impulses strike the cell membrane, travel down the T tubules, and cause calcium release.

When a muscle cell receives an electrical impulse, it responds by contracting. Here's how: Once stimulated, the cell's membrane becomes increasingly permeable to sodium. Sodium ions enter the cell, causing the cell to depolarize and potassium to leave. Calcium then moves into the cell through slow channels.

Free calcium ions bind to troponin, which alters tropomyosin's configuration. This allows actin and myosin to interact and form cross-bridges of electrochemical activity. As they do, the cardiac muscle shortens and contracts.

During final repolarization, troponin and tropomyosin resume their roles as actin-myosin inhibitors. Actin filaments slide away from each other and from the myosin filaments. The cardiac muscle then lengthens and relaxes.

Myocardial muscle fiber

This cross section of sarcoplasmic reticulum covering the myocardial muscle fibers reveals a myofibril, composed of thick myosin and thin actin filaments.

The detailed segment below it shows dark A bands of myosin and lighter I bands of actin. The sarcomere serves as the muscle cell's contractile unit.

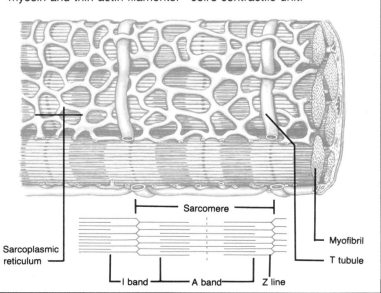

Sarcoplasmic reticulum
Sarcomere
Myofibril
T tubule
I band — A band — Z line

Muscle Dysfunction

What causes heart failure. Heart failure sometimes develops in a patient with normal heart function, from an imbalance between the body's metabolic needs and the volume of blood pumped by the heart.

In newborns, infants, and children, congenital heart disease most frequently causes heart failure. Structural abnormalities such as ventricular septal defect, transposition of the great vessels, aortic atresia, coarctation of the aorta, and patent ductus arteriosus strain the heart hemodynamically.

In adults, heart failure usually stems from conditions causing abnormal volume or pressure load on the heart, abnormal muscle function, or unusual metabolic demands by body tissues. To understand why, let's examine each cause.

Continued on page 64

Tracking the cardiac cycle

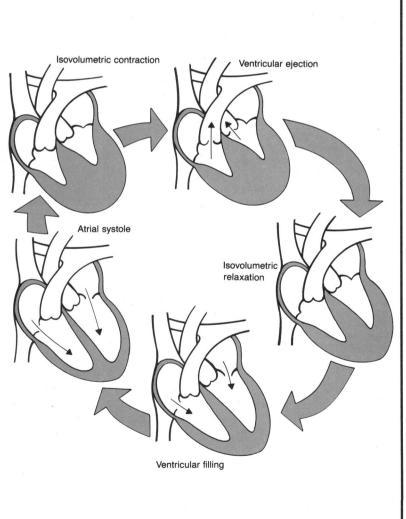

Cardiac cycle refers to ventricular diastole and systole (unless otherwise specified). *Isovolumetric ventricular contraction* begins the cycle. Responding to ventricular depolarization, the ventricles contract. The resulting pressure increase leads to mitral and tricuspid valve closure. Thus, all four valves remain closed for this short time (the pulmonic and aortic valves stay closed during this entire phase).

In *ventricular ejection*, the next phase, ventricular pressure exceeds aortic and pulmonary arterial pressure. The aortic and pulmonic valves open, permitting ejection of ventricular blood.

Ventricular pressure now drops below that of the aorta and pulmonary artery, signalling the *isovolumetric relaxation phase*. This causes aortic and pulmonic valve closure, so all four valves again remain closed. (*Note:* Atrial diastole occurs now as blood fills the atria.)

During *ventricular filling*, atrial pressure exceeds ventricular pressure. This in turn triggers mitral and tricuspid valve opening, permitting passive blood flow into the ventricles. About 80% of ventricular filling now takes place.

Atrial systole, the last phase, coincides with late diastole, when the atria contract in response to atrial depolarization. This "atrial kick" supplies the ventricles with the remaining 20% of blood.

And the cycle repeats...

Muscle Dysfunction

Defining some important terms

Cardiac output (CO) refers to the volume of blood ejected by the heart each minute. Cardiac output normally ranges from 4 to 8 liters. In ordinary conditions, the heart pumps only as much blood as it needs. When needs change, the heart adjusts its output.

Stroke volume (SV) (see below) and *heart rate (HR)* determine cardiac output, as expressed in this formula: $CO = SV \times HR$.

Stroke volume refers to the difference between volume at the end of diastole (EDV) (just before the heart contracts), and volume in the left ventricle at the end of systole (ESV).

Three factors determine stroke volume: *preload*, *afterload*, and *contractility*.

Preload, the ventricular volume plus pressure at diastole's end, determines muscle fiber length when contraction begins. This length in turn determines contractile force and the velocity of muscle fiber shortening.

Afterload means the impedance, or resistance, the ventricle works against to eject blood during systole. Impedance hinges on arterial blood pressure, valve characteristics, and ventricular radius and wall thickness.

Contractility refers to the ventricle's contractile ability. Myocardial contraction force and/or the extent of muscle fiber shortening depend on initial muscle length. Muscle fibers lengthen, within limits, in response to increased stretch, ejecting larger amounts of blood with greater force.

Heart rate also affects cardiac output. If stroke volume decreases, heart rate will increase to maintain cardiac output. Sinoatrial (SA) node automaticity and the autonomic nervous system influence heart rate. Parasympathetic nerves release acetylcholine, which depresses SA node automaticity, slows conduction through the AV (atrioventricular) junction, and decreases heart rate. Sympathetic nerves release norepinephrine, which enhances SA node automaticity, increases AV junction conduction, strengthens myocardial contractility, and increases heart rate.

Heart failure—*continued*

Volume or pressure load increase. When conditions such as hypertension and aortic or pulmonic stenosis place excessive pressure demands on the ventricle, this chamber must in turn generate enough pressure to overcome the load and open the semilunar valve. Generating this pressure for a prolonged time can strain the heart.

Meanwhile, the myocardium may compensate for the increased load by increasing its muscle mass. Initially, this may improve contractility, but eventually, hypertrophied tissue interferes with ventricular functioning. If ventricular pressure remains high, the heart may begin to fail.

Similarly, increasing ventricular volume may strain the heart chambers. Blood regurgitating across a leaking or incompetent valve causes increased volume. Other conditions that cause volume overload include ventricular septal defects, atrial septal defects, patent ductus arteriosus, and lesions allowing shunting of blood between chambers.

How well the heart tolerates the volume increase depends on the amount of increase and how quickly the increase develops. Small volume increases stretch myocardial cells and subsequently strengthen contractions—a compensatory response, known as Starling's law. If volume overload increases further, a second compensatory mechanism comes into play—ventricular dilation. The enlargement allows ventricular pressures to remain normal. Ventricular hypertrophy may also occur, helping to strengthen contractions.

Generally, the body tolerates slow, progressive volume increases better than abrupt ones. A sudden increase in ventricular volume allows no time for compensatory dilation. A normal-size ventricle receiving a sudden volume increase can't accommodate the excess. Consequently, ventricular pressure rises sharply and heart failure ensues.

Abnormal muscle function. If muscle cells can't adequately contract and relax, the heart can't pump efficiently. In adults, myocardial infarction (MI) accounts for most heart muscle dysfunction. Irreversible myocardial damage creates an area of nonfunctioning ventricular muscle cells. Depending on the extent of the necrosis, pump function may suffer.

Other forms of intrinsic myocardial disease include inflammatory processes such as infectious myocarditis, rheumatic heart disease, and systemic lupus erythematosus, as well as cardiomyopathies. Although each disease process affects the heart differently, all may alter myocardial cell performance so that overall ventricular function suffers.

In addition to myocardial cell abnormalities, other conditions may impair normal myocardial function. External factors such as pericardial effusion, cardiac tamponade, and constrictive pericarditis adversely affect ventricular filling during diastole. As a result, the ventricles can't fill or empty adequately, and cardiac function falters.

Muscle Dysfunction

Compensatory mechanisms that help maintain normal cardiac pumping

• The Frank-Starling mechanism refers to the relationship between preload and myocardial contraction strength. As preload increases, contractility increases and sustains cardiac output.

• An increased catecholamine release augments myocardial contractility.

• Myocardial hypertrophy—with or without cardiac chamber dilatation—augments contractile tissue mass, thus improving contractility.

Increased metabolic demands. Conditions such as severe anemia, thyrotoxicosis, pregnancy, fever, and sepsis can trigger an imbalance between the heart's ability to supply oxygen and the body's oxygen demand. This results in high-output failure (explained later).

Compensatory mechanisms and medications help control chronic heart failure. However, several conditions may upset the balance between pump function and oxygen demand—most commonly dysrhythmias. By causing extreme rate, rhythm, and conduction disturbances, dysrhythmias impair the heart's ability to fill with and eject blood, reduce cardiac perfusion, increase oxygen needs, and generally diminish pumping efficiency. When this occurs, cardiac output drops. To a patient with compromised cardiac function, this sudden change in pumping action poses a grave threat. Unless controlled, dysrhythmias may trigger symptomatic heart failure.

How heart failure progresses. Typically, heart failure begins in the left ventricle. When this ventricle fails to eject sufficient blood, baroreceptors in the aorta and other areas cause reflex stimulation of the sympathetic nervous system. As a result:
• veins and venules constrict, increasing blood return to the heart
• arteries and arterioles constrict, maintaining systemic blood pressure and redistributing blood away from nonvital areas
• contractility increases, directly affecting myocardial cells and producing stronger contractions
• heart rate increases from sympathetic receptors that affect pacemaker cells.

These changes also curb blood flow to the kidneys. Special cells in the kidneys' arterioles detect the decrease and release renin. This stimulates the renin-angiotensin-aldosterone system, leading to vasoconstriction and sodium and water retention. Initially, this compensatory mechanism helps restore cardiac output by increasing blood pressure, augmenting blood volume, and generally improving venous return to the heart.

But when heart failure progresses despite compensation, decompensation begins. As the heart beats faster, it demands more oxygen. But a faster heart rate also shortens diastole, reducing ventricular filling time. As a result, the left ventricle supplies even less oxygenated blood to the coronary arteries.

As heart failure progresses, peripheral vasoconstriction, which helped protect vital organs during compensation, contributes to decompensation. Vasoconstriction increases vascular resistance in turn, forcing the failing heart to pump even harder.

The renin-angiotensin-aldosterone system may also promote decompensation by overfilling the heart. As compensatory mechanisms eventually fail, volume overload leads to increased ventricular pressure.

Heart failure constitutes a vicious cycle—left ventricular failure progresses from a compensated to a decompensated state. Left heart failure then leads to right heart failure.

Continued on page 66

Muscle Dysfunction

Heart failure—*continued*

Common heart failure terms

You may hear various terms used to describe heart failure. This quick review will help you distinguish them.

High-output vs. low-output failure. When conditions such as CAD, hypertension, valvular heart disease, and cardiomyopathy impair pump function and slow blood flow to healthy tissue, low-output pump failure (the most common type) results. As mentioned earlier, high-output failure occurs when diseased tissue demands more blood than even a healthy heart can supply. High-output failure may result from anemia, thyrotoxicosis, or pregnancy.

Both high-output and low-output failure impair oxygen delivery to the tissues. Although treatment of the two types may differ, the goal remains controlling the primary cause of the oxygen supply and demand imbalance.

Forward vs. backward failure. When pump inefficiency causes increased volume and pressure in the affected ventricle and atrium, pressure also builds in the venous bed behind the ventricle. As this happens, fluid moves from the capillary bed to the interstitial space, and congestive signs and symptoms arise. This "backward failure" theory implies that in left ventricular failure, blood accumulation and congestion take place in the pulmonary system. If blood builds

---

The route to congestive heart failure

In left heart failure, increased work load and end-diastolic volume enlarges the left ventricle. This diminishes left ventricular function, allowing blood to pool in the ventricle and atrium. Eventually, blood backs up into pulmonary veins and capillaries, leading to elevated capillary pressure. In response, sodium and water enter the interstitial space, resulting in pulmonary edema.

As vascular pressure increases and left cardiac function decreases, the right ventricle shows signs of stress such as hypertrophy, increased conduction time, and dysrhythmias.

When the patient lies down, pulmonary edema worsens because excess fluid from the legs pools in the pulmonary circulation.

Blood pools in the right ventricle and atrium, causing pressure and congestion in the vena cava and elevating general circulation. Backed-up blood also distends visceral veins, and the liver and spleen become engorged. In response to rising capillary pressure, capillary fluid flows into the interstitial space. This causes tissue edema, especially in the lower legs and abdomen.

Muscle Dysfunction

up in the right side, however, fluid will accumulate in systemic areas such as the liver, abdomen, and extremities. This theory hinges on the concept that although each ventricle may fail independently, failure of one usually triggers failure of the other.

The theory of forward failure asserts that heart failure's effects remain secondary to the heart's inability to maintain forward flow. Poor perfusion to vital organs such as the brain, kidneys, liver, and skeletal muscles accounts for many heart failure signs and symptoms.

Because both forward and backward theories seem valid, they've generated controversy for years. But researchers now accept both theories as a dual mechanism in most heart failure patients.

Although some patients can have isolated forward or backward failure, most have signs and symptoms of both. These findings frequently go by the term congestive heart failure (CHF).

Right vs. left heart failure. Like backward failure, right and left heart failure involve fluid accumulation behind the affected ventricle. But here the similarity ends. Right heart failure produces systemic effects, whereas left heart failure produces primarily pulmonary effects.

Acute vs. chronic failure. How quickly heart failure develops determines when signs and symptoms appear and how well the patient tolerates them. He may tolerate chronic or slowly developing failure for years through compensation, while failure of sudden onset bars compensation. Thus, patient care focuses on preventing chronic failure from progressing to acute failure. Such disorders as dysrhythmias and volume overload can upset the delicate balance maintained by the medical, dietary, and exercise regimen of a patient with chronic failure.

Assessment

When assessing a patient with possible heart failure, consider his health history, chief complaints, symptoms, and physical signs. This information helps you gauge the problem's severity and identify the involved heart chambers.

In most cases, heart failure findings result from expanding blood volume, pulmonary and systemic vascular bed congestion, and excessive sodium and water retention. As a general rule, expect pulmonary signs and symptoms with left heart failure, and systemic signs and symptoms with right heart failure. But keep in mind that heart failure frequently affects both sides.

Left heart failure signs and symptoms. Expect dyspnea at rest or on exertion. The patient may describe dyspnea as breathlessness, breathing difficulty, or shortness of breath. (Dyspnea's usually noted first on exertion.) The patient may catch his breath in mid-sentence. Because dyspnea usually eases with rest, the patient may initially dismiss this symptom as minor. But as heart failure progresses, dyspnea may also appear during rest.

Continued on page 68

Muscle Dysfunction

Heart failure—*continued*

In addition, your patient may suffer orthopnea (dyspnea occurring while lying down) and paroxysmal nocturnal dyspnea (dyspnea occurring after a few hours sleep). These dyspnea types may occur because the supine position increases venous return to the heart, adding to fluid overload. Sitting upright relieves symptoms.

Expect to hear crackles (rales) in the lung fields—a result of pulmonary congestion—possibly accompanied by wheezes (rhonchi).

Vague signs and symptoms such as fatigue, weakness, and nocturia may also accompany left heart failure, as decreased cardiac output causes poor oxygen and blood delivery to the skeletal muscles. The patient may also complain of intermittent or constant heaviness in his arms or legs.

Increased pulmonary pressure and bronchial tree edema may cause a nonproductive, dry cough. Sputum, if present, usually appears scanty and clear.

Right heart failure signs and symptoms. Check for indications of dependent peripheral edema, such as swollen feet or ankles. A patient confined to bed may have sacral edema. To identify any edema, ask these questions: Do your clothes fit more tightly than before? Do your shoes leave a mark or feel snug? Do your rings feel tighter than normal? Such changes suggest right heart failure.

Other indications include organ engorgement, especially of the liver and spleen; jugular vein distention; and ascites. The patient may report a slow weight gain of 10 to 15 lb (4.5 to 6.8 kg). Accumulating fluid may also bring on a feeling of abdominal fullness or pain, nausea, and loss of appetite. You may also note tachycardia, distended neck veins, abdominal tenderness or enlargement, and hepatojugular reflux.

Remember, signs and symptoms of heart failure vary depending on the degree of compensation and the failure's severity. Carefully evaluate the patient's description of his symptoms, keeping in mind that his viewpoint's subjective. Use objective physical findings such as crackles, wheezes, edema, ascites, cyanosis, and abnormal heart sounds to help pinpoint the problem.

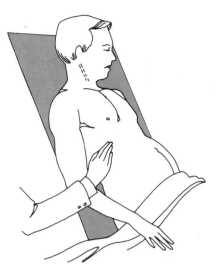

If you suspect right ventricular heart failure in your patient, assess for hepatojugular reflux. Firmly and slowly compress the patient's abdomen over the liver (see the illustration above). If he has right heart failure, this action will increase the forward flow of blood to the right atrium, elevating jugular venous pressure and distending jugular veins.

Heart failure: Signs and symptoms

As a rule, expect pulmonary signs and symptoms in left heart failure; systemic signs and symptoms in right heart failure. Read the following for details on how signs and symptoms differ.

Left heart failure	Right heart failure
• Elevated blood pressure • Paroxysmal nocturnal dyspnea, dyspnea on exertion, orthopnea • Bronchial wheezing • Hypoxia, respiratory acidosis • Crackles • Cough with frothy pink sputum • Cyanosis or pallor • Third or fourth heart sounds • Palpitations, dysrhythmias • Elevated pulmonary artery diastolic and pulmonary capillary wedge pressures • Pulsus alternans	• Weakness, fatigue, dizziness, syncope • Hepatomegaly, with or without pain • Ascites • Dependent pitting peripheral edema • Jugular vein distention • Hepatojugular reflux • Oliguria • Dysrhythmias • Elevated central venous/right atrial pressure • Nausea, vomiting, anorexia, abdominal distention • Weight gain

Muscle Dysfunction

Measuring cardiac output and determining cardiac index

You can use the thermodilution technique to determine cardiac output if your patient has a pulmonary (PA) catheter equipped with a thermistor.

First connect the catheter's thermistor hub to a cardiac output computer. Inject the indicator solution (usually cold normal saline solution or dextrose 5% in water) into the catheter's proximal lumen. The indicator solution mixes with blood in the heart's right side. As this blood flows past the catheter's distal end, the thermistor detects the temperature change. The computer analyzes this information and records the patient's cardiac output on a display screen. (*Note:* You can also use room-temperature solution; however, be sure to adjust computer settings accordingly.) Normally, cardiac output measures 4 to 8 liters/min. By calculating cardiac index, which takes body size into account, you can find out whether your patient's cardiac output meets his needs. Cardiac index normally ranges from 2.5 to 4.2 liters/min/m².

To calculate cardiac index, first calculate the patient's body surface area using a nomogram. To do this, find his height (left column) and his weight (right column). Using a ruler, connect these two points. You'll find his body surface area at the point where the ruler intersects the center column.

Now calculate your patient's cardiac index using the formula below.

Cardiac index =

$$\frac{\text{Cardiac output (liter/min)}}{\text{Body surface area (m}^2)}$$

Diagnostic studies. No single diagnostic test conclusively proves heart failure. To confirm the condition and gauge its severity, type, and cause, the doctor will weigh findings from the patient's history, physical examination, and laboratory studies, including arterial blood gas measurements (ABGs) and chest X-ray. ABGs may show mildly decreased PaO_2 with normal or decreased $PaCO_2$. Severe failure frequently brings on metabolic acidosis. A chest X-ray may show cardiac dilatation from compensatory changes and may detect any pleural effusion. It may also reveal pulmonary vein and artery prominence from high pulmonary pressure. As congestion increases, densities and haziness appear in areas of fluid accumulation—usually both bases.

Routine laboratory findings vary according to the degree of failure and any treatment the patient's received. If failure affects the patient's renal function, his blood urea nitrogen levels may increase. Excessive diuretic use can lead to a low serum potassium level. With right heart failure, expect abnormal findings in liver function studies.

Continued on page 70

How heart failure affects circulation

Right heart failure
Impaired right pump function (see darker area below) reduces cardiac output. Although systemic venous pressures rise, the body compensates to maintain pulmonary artery and left ventricular end-diastolic pressures at normal levels.

Left heart failure
When the left pump fails (see lighter area below), cardiac output drops. Increased left ventricular end-diastolic pressure elevates pulmonary venous pressures, but compensatory mechanisms maintain mean aortic pressures at normal levels. Increased pulmonary venous pressure also increases pulmonary artery pressure.

Biventricular congestive heart failure
In moderately severe heart failure (includes both areas below), cardiac output falls; pulmonary venous pressure, pulmonary artery pressure, and systemic venous pressures rise. As cardiac output drops, mean arterial pressure decreases.

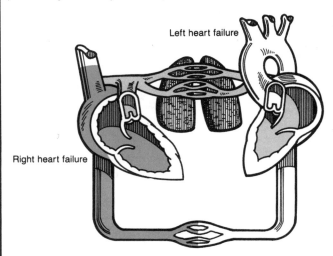

Left heart failure

Right heart failure

Muscle Dysfunction

Heart failure—*continued*

Although an EKG won't specifically reveal heart failure, it can demonstrate compensatory tachycardia as well as MI. In a patient with chronic heart failure, an EKG may show ventricular or atrial enlargement. Echocardiography may give clues to failure's underlying causes, although it can't specifically show the disorder.

A central venous pressure (CVP) or pulmonary artery (PA) catheter helps estimate the degree of failure and the patient's response to treatment. CVP, which reflects right heart function, may be normal or mildly elevated in left heart failure. In right heart failure, CVP shows a marked increase.

The PA line measures pulmonary arterial pressure and can help evaluate left ventricular function. Pressure increases in left heart failure. In pure right heart failure, it may be low or normal.

Nuclear studies may help pinpoint heart failure's causes. (For more information on diagnostic tests, see Chapter 2.)

Planning

Nursing diagnosis. Base your nursing diagnosis for a heart failure patient on his clinical condition. Before formulating a care plan, determine the patient's actual or potential problems. To determine the nursing diagnosis, relate these problems to their cause. Possible nursing diagnoses for the heart failure patient include the following:
• cardiac output, alteration in (decreased); related to increased ventricular volume and filling pressure
• fluid volume, alteration in (excess); related to decreased pumping ability
• anxiety; related to illness
• activity intolerance; related to fatigue and dyspnea
• gas exchange, impaired; related to pulmonary congestion
• sleep pattern disturbance; related to dyspnea, nocturia
• tissue perfusion, alteration in; related to decreased cardiac output
• skin integrity, impairment of (potential); related to immobility
• knowledge deficit; related to disease process
• noncompliance (potential); related to inadequate health teaching
• family processes, alteration in; related to disease.

The box on page 71 shows a sample nursing care plan for a heart failure patient based on one nursing diagnosis. But remember to adapt your care plan to the needs of your patient and his family. (*Note:* The generalized care plan shown presents a sample listing of expected outcomes, nursing interventions, and discharge planning that may apply to your patient.)

Intervention

Although acute and chronic heart failure may produce different signs and symptoms, the basic treatment goal remains the same: to reverse the compensatory-decompensatory cycle, thus maximizing cardiac function.

Muscle Dysfunction

Sample nursing care plan—Chronic congestive heart failure

Nursing diagnosis	Expected outcomes
Cardiac output, alteration in (decreased); related to increased ventricular volume and filling pressure	The patient will: • maintain adequate cardiac output and perfusion • have little or no edema or weight gain • perform his ADL with little fatigue or dyspnea • show knowledge of the rationale for his care plan and treatment • show knowledge of how to prevent or reduce alterations in cardiac output.
Nursing interventions • Observe for signs and symptoms of decreased cardiac output and perfusion. • Monitor vital signs for indications of increasing pulmonic or systemic venous congestion. • Maintain adequate fluid intake and output. • Provide low-sodium diet. • Auscultate heart for S_3 and S_4. • Auscultate lungs for crackles and wheezes. • Provide frequent rest periods. • Elevate patient's feet when he's out of bed. • Discuss purpose of treatment and care plan with patient, teaching him about his medications and diet. • Monitor medication effects. • Provide information on and maintain activities that reduce the heart's work load. • Give emotional support. • Discuss strategies to help him perform his ADL with little fatigue or dyspnea.	**Discharge planning** • Teach patient about his medications. • Reinforce treatment plan and patient's need to comply. • Teach patient when to seek medical care. • Discuss with patient—and his family or support persons—ways to modify his ADL to reduce fatigue, dyspnea, and edema.

To do this, the doctor will attempt to remove heart failure's underlying or precipitating causes with therapies that:
• improve pump performance through digitalis or positive inotropic drug therapy
• reduce cardiac work load through vasodilator therapy, anxiety reduction, rest, assisted circulation, or weight reduction
• control salt and water retention through diuretics, a low-sodium diet, or mechanical fluid removal.

Drug therapy. Inotropes, diuretics, and vasodilators can quickly and markedly reduce cardiac work load.

Inotropes. These drugs maximize cardiac performance by increasing ventricular contractility. Digoxin, an oral inotropic, increases intracellular calcium at the cell membrane, permitting stronger contractions. It also produces electrophysiologic changes that decrease AV nodal conduction. These effects, together with improved cardiac output, help decrease heart rate in a CHF patient. As cardiac output improves, the heart no longer needs to maintain tachycardia to compensate for poor pumping action.

Check the patient's apical and radial pulse rates before administering digoxin; report significant pulse changes to the doctor. Also closely observe the patient's serum electrolyte levels; digoxin could irritate his heart if his potassium level's low.

Continued on page 72

Muscle Dysfunction

Unlike digitalis glycosides and catecholamines, *amrinone lactate* (a cardiac inotropic drug) increases the force and velocity of myocardial systolic contraction and dilates peripheral vessels. The drug usually increases cardiac output quickly without significantly changing heart rate or blood pressure. Because amrinone adds to digitalis' effects, it can be given to a fully digitalized patient without causing cardiac glycoside toxicity.

The doctor may order amrinone lactate for short-term management of congestive heart failure in patients unresponsive to digitalis, diuretic, and vasodilator therapy.

When administering this drug, stay alert for adverse effects such as thrombocytopenia, dysrhythmias, hypotension, nausea, vomiting, hepatotoxicity, and hypersensitivity reactions.

Initial therapy calls for 0.75 mg/kg bolus given slowly over 2 to 3 min, followed by an infusion of 5 to 10 mcg/kg/min. Another 0.75 mg/kg bolus may be given 30 min after therapy starts. The usual total daily dose shouldn't exceed 10 mg/kg.

Always give amrinone either as supplied or diluted in normal or half-normal saline solution to a concentration of 1 to 3 mg/ml. Don't dilute the drug with solutions containing dextrose, because a slow chemical reaction will occur. But you can inject amrinone into infusing dextrose. Be sure to monitor the patient's heart rate and measure his blood pressure during administration. If his vital signs change, slow or stop the infusion. Monitor potassium levels and measure intake and output.

Still under study, *milrinone*, an amrinone derivative, appears to enhance contractility and peripheral vasodilation. Milrinone has almost 20 times amrinone's inotropic potency, but doesn't seem to cause thrombocytopenia and fever.

Heart failure—*continued*

Stay alert for signs and symptoms of digoxin toxicity such as anorexia, nausea, vomiting, and visual disturbances. Also check for interactions with other medication by monitoring serum digoxin levels. Neomycin, Kaopectate, and some antacids decrease GI digoxin absorption. Antiarrhythmics such as quinidine and verapamil can elevate serum digoxin levels.

For a patient with acute congestive heart failure, the doctor may order I.V. administration of dopamine, dobutamine, or the new drug amrinone. These drugs improve the heart's pumping ability. Depending on the drug and dose used, they may also dilate the vessels, which reduces cardiac work load by decreasing pump pressure. The combined positive inotropy and vasodilation help "unload" the failing heart.

Diuretics. By increasing urinary output, these drugs help reduce cardiac preload. Available in both oral and parenteral form, diuretics vary greatly in mechanism and site of action, potency, and adverse effects. Diuretics that act in the kidney's proximal tubule generally produce fewer benefits because other kidney sites may reverse their effects. Thiazide and potassium-sparing diuretics act on the proximal and distal convoluted tubules to produce more efficient diuresis.

Loop diuretics, the most potent, interfere with chloride reabsorption at Henle's loop. They improve cardiac function by decreasing volume load. Commonly used loop diuretics include Lasix, Edecrin, and Bumex.

These potent drugs can produce more severe adverse effects than other diuretics. Excessive use may cause dehydration, taking the patient from one extreme (volume overload) to the other (volume depletion). If potassium stores diminish, electrolyte imbalance may result. To prevent this life-threatening effect, monitor serum potassium levels and supplement potassium, as needed.

The doctor will probably use conservative diuretic therapy initially. If appropriate, he'll increase the dose or order a different diuretic type. Milder diuretics such as thiazide may alleviate the patient's signs and symptoms while reducing the risk of volume depletion and dehydration; however, even mild diuretics can deplete potassium stores. To avoid this, consider giving dietary or other potassium supplements.

Potassium-sparing diuretics, such as spironolactone, amiloride, and triamterene, act in the kidneys' distal tubules. These drugs work best when used with other diuretics. Use extreme care when giving these drugs to a patient with severe CHF or renal dysfunction, as they may cause metabolic acidosis and hyperkalemia.

Vasodilators. The doctor may order vasodilators to augment inotropes and diuretics. Vasodilators come in three types: venodilators, arteriodilators, and mixed (which dilate arterioles and veins).

Venodilators, including nitroglycerin and other nitrates, directly relax smooth muscles by producing generalized dilation that affects veins more than arteries. They decrease venous return to the heart.

Muscle Dysfunction

Arteriodilators, including hydralazine, minoxidil, and nifedipine, act principally on arterioles. They diminish cardiac work load by decreasing peripheral vascular resistance. They also increase renal and cerebral blood flow.

Mixed vasodilators, such as nitroprusside, prazosin, and captopril, improve cardiac output by facilitating ventricular emptying and reducing peripheral vascular resistance, thus decreasing myocardial oxygen demand.

Oxygen therapy. Your patient may need supplemental oxygen in addition to drugs.

Fluid removal. A patient with chronic heart failure may require excess cardiac fluid removal through thoracentesis, paracentesis, or rarely, dialysis.

Mechanical devices. A patient with severe, poorly controlled heart failure may need a mechanical device to maintain cardiac function. Such devices especially suit the patient with a reparable defect such as severe CAD, ventricular aneurysm, or a defective valve. The intraaortic balloon pump (IABP), the most commonly used device for heart failure, helps sustain a patient until surgical correction (such as valve repair or heart transplantation) becomes feasible. It also helps maintain cardiac function during and just after surgery in a patient who's had cardiopulmonary bypass.

Continued on page 74

A mechanical boost for the failing heart

Artificial hearts
Still investigational, artificial hearts have been transplanted in several patients. The Jarvik-7, the most well-known, takes its name from its designer, Robert Jarvik, MD. The device consists of two mechanical ventricles attached to Dacron sleeves sewn to the patient's aorta, pulmonary artery, and atria. Compressed air activates the internal diaphragm and valves and powers the heart, which doctors connect to a drive unit. The artificial heart then functions as the patient's own.

Other artificial hearts under investigation include the Penn State and Phoenix hearts.

Ventricular assist devices (VADs)
These investigational devices augment heart action in patients with inadequate cardiac pump function. A VAD may serve as a temporary support for a patient awaiting heart transplantation or who can't be weaned from a heart-lung machine. These devices may eventually provide an alternative to the artificial heart.

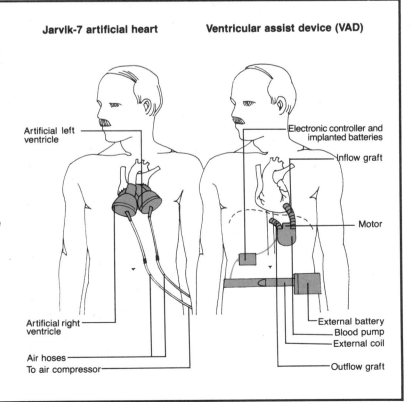

Jarvik-7 artificial heart
- Artificial left ventricle
- Artificial right ventricle
- Air hoses
- To air compressor

Ventricular assist device (VAD)
- Electronic controller and implanted batteries
- Inflow graft
- Motor
- External battery
- Blood pump
- External coil
- Outflow graft

Muscle Dysfunction

Intraaortic balloon pump (IABP)

Also known as intraaortic balloon counterpulsation (IABC), the IABP augments coronary artery blood flow, permitting more oxygen and nutrients to reach the heart.

The IABP best treats patients with cardiogenic shock, pump failure, mechanical MI complications, and unstable angina resistant to medical treatment. It can also serve as a circulatory assist before heart transplantation. Contraindications for IABP include irreversible brain damage, chronic end-stage heart disease, incompetent aortic valve, aortic or thoracic aneurysm, and peripheral vascular disease.

The doctor usually inserts the balloon catheter into the aorta by way of the femoral artery. The console determines inflation and deflation cycles according to the patient's EKG or arterial waveform.

Inflated with helium or carbon dioxide during diastole, the balloon increases aortic diastolic pressure, which in turn enhances coronary blood flow and perfusion.

During systole, the balloon deflates, permitting the left ventricle to eject blood into the aorta at a lower pressure.

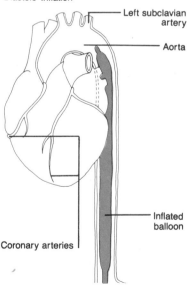

Diastole Inflation

— Left subclavian artery

— Aorta

— Inflated balloon

Coronary arteries

Heart failure—*continued*

The doctor inserts the intraaortic balloon percutaneously through the femoral artery and into the descending aorta, slightly beyond the origin of the left subclavian artery. The balloon inflates and deflates in synchrony with cardiac events. Inflation, which occurs during diastole, increases aortic pressure and improves coronary artery blood flow. Deflation, occurring at the onset of systole, lowers aortic pressure and ventricular resistance. The resulting increase in coronary artery perfusion and decrease in ventricular resistance lead to a drop in myocardial oxygen demand and to increased cardiac output.

Left ventricular assist devices (LVADs) and implantable artificial hearts, now under investigation, may also help treat heart failure. The LVAD diverts blood from the left ventricle to the ascending aorta, reducing left ventricular work load and maintaining circulation. Patients with severe CHF after cardiac surgery, cardiogenic shock, and cardiomyopathy have used LVADs—some for weeks at a time.

A totally implantable artificial heart such as the Jarvik-7 has two mechanical ventricles that attach to the patient's aorta, pulmonary artery, and atria. Compressed air activates the device's diaphragms and valves to circulate blood through the lungs and body. Still experimental, artificial heart implantation takes place only at a few medical centers. Most patients receiving these implants have had irreversible heart disease.

For some patients with irreversible heart disease, heart transplantation offers another option. For information on this procedure, see page 78.

Complications

Pulmonary edema and cardiogenic shock commonly complicate heart failure. Pulmonary edema generally develops when left heart failure progresses, leading to extreme pulmonary vessel pressure that forces fluid from the vascular space into lung interstitium. The resulting pulmonary congestion advances depending on the heart's work load and ventricular function.

Signs and symptoms of pulmonary edema mimic those of congestive heart failure but seem more severe. Check for air hunger, suffocation, and extreme apprehension. Unable to lie flat, the patient may try to sit upright to improve oxygenation. Expect tachypnea and labored breathing. You may hear crackles or wheezes without a stethoscope.

Hypoxia and decreased cardiac output may make the patient restless, pale, ashen, cool, and diaphoretic. His vital signs will depend on the degree of cardiac compromise. Without intervention, pulmonary edema can rapidly lead to marked hypotension, cardiogenic shock, and death. Treatment aims at reducing fluid volume and improving oxygenation.

In Stage I pulmonary edema, the chest's lymphatic system drains fluid away from the interstitial space. Signs and symptoms may occur only with exertion, although a chest X-ray may indicate the problem.

Muscle Dysfunction

If your patient's heart failure deteriorates to pulmonary edema, intervene quickly and efficiently, according to these guidelines:
• **Call for help.** Notify the doctor at once and gather emergency equipment.
• **Assess and ensure airway patency and oxygenation.** Maintain proper airway position. Encourage coughing, if it's productive. Suction only if absolutely necessary to avoid further decreasing oxygen levels. Administer oxygen by mask or nasal cannula. Prepare for IPPB treatment if ordered, and for drawing of ABGs.
• **Position the patient to decrease venous return.** If possible, place him in high Fowler's position, letting his legs dangle to further decrease venous return. Monitor blood pressure closely.
• **Assess vital signs routinely.** Check his vital signs frequently until his condition stabilizes.
• **Start an I.V..** Choose an insertion site unaffected by position changes.
• **Attach cardiac monitor.** Observe closely for dysrhythmias.
• **Administer medications as ordered.** Prepare to give Lasix, morphine, and digoxin I.V. as ordered. The doctor may also order other medications such as nitroglycerin, nitroprusside, and dobutamine.
• **Prepare rotating tourniquets if needed.** This technique pools blood in three extremities at once, decreasing venous return to the overloaded heart. *Important:* Don't use this method with a hypotensive patient.
• **Calculate strict fluid intake and output.** Be prepared to insert an indwelling (Foley) catheter, if ordered, to monitor intake and output. Restrict fluids.
• **Prepare resuscitation equipment.** Have advanced life support equipment on hand and keep intubation supplies in the patient's room.
• **Provide emotional support.** Maintain a calm, caring attitude. Reassure the patient and his family. Remain with the patient as much as possible and provide the family with a quiet waiting area.

Stage II pulmonary edema occurs when interstitial fluid accumulates faster than the lymphatic system can drain it. Edema develops in bronchioles, venules, and arteries. As oxygen needs increase, dyspnea, orthopnea, and paroxysmal nocturnal dyspnea arise. Suspect this edema type if the patient has tachypnea, cough, apprehension, and fine, crepitant crackles over both lung bases.

Alveolar edema, the hallmark of Stage III pulmonary edema, develops from excessive pulmonary pressure and rapid fluid transudation from vascular and interstitial spaces into alveoli. Surrounded by fluid and high pressure, alveoli collapse, which dramatically impairs oxygen exchange.

Cardiogenic shock stems from severe circulatory failure resulting from impaired pumping ability. This condition frequently follows an acute MI—especially one that damages 40% or more of the left ventricle. Cardiogenic shock may also occur with end-stage cardiomyopathy or a mechanical defect such as valve rupture, ventricular septal defect, or tamponade.

Because cardiogenic shock results from a marked decrease in functional ventricular muscle tissue, watch for signs and symptoms of decreased cardiac output, such as restlessness, confusion, diaphoresis, cold, clammy skin, rapid and thready pulse, and diminished urinary output. Depending on the patient's volume status, left ventricular failure or pulmonary edema may also appear. When car-

Continued on page 76

Picturing pulmonary edema

The left ventricle's diminished function causes blood to pool in the left ventricle and atrium, eventually backing up into the pulmonary veins and capillaries. Rising capillary hydrostatic pressure pushes fluid into the interstitial spaces and alveoli.

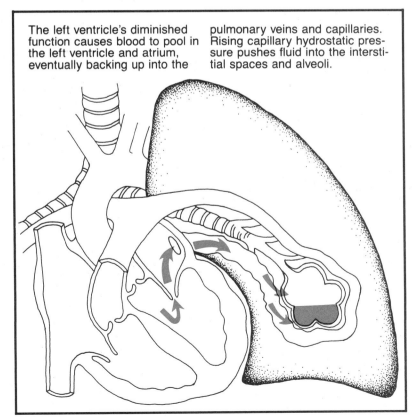

Muscle Dysfunction

Cardiogenic shock: A decompensation cycle

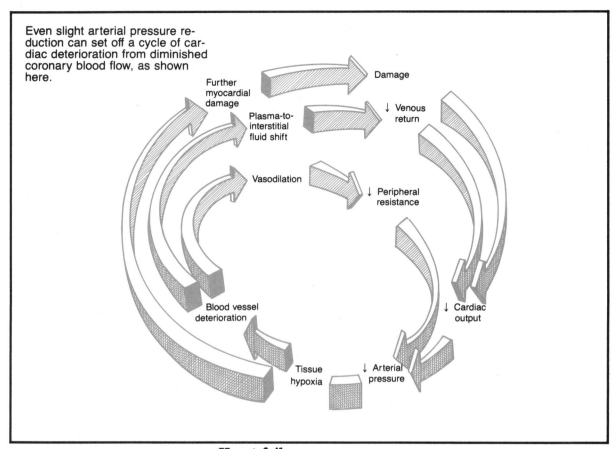

Even slight arterial pressure reduction can set off a cycle of cardiac deterioration from diminished coronary blood flow, as shown here.

Further myocardial damage

Damage

Plasma-to-interstitial fluid shift

↓ Venous return

Vasodilation

↓ Peripheral resistance

Blood vessel deterioration

↓ Cardiac output

Tissue hypoxia

↓ Arterial pressure

Heart failure—*continued*

diogenic shock stems from a mechanical defect, the IABP helps stabilize the patient until surgery can correct the defect. But when shock results from extensive myocardial damage, the patient may become dependent on the IABP because existing muscle tissue can't sustain sufficient cardiac output.

Evaluation

Base your evaluation on the patient's expected outcomes listed on your nursing care plan. To determine if his condition's improved, ask yourself these questions:
• Can he maintain adequate cardiac output and perfusion?
• Does he show excessive edema or weight gain?
• Can he perform daily activities without dyspnea or excessive fatigue?
• Does he understand his care plan and treatment?
• Does he know how to prevent or reduce alterations in cardiac output?

The answers to these questions will help you evaluate your patient's status and the effectiveness of his care. Keep in mind that these questions stem from the care plan shown on page 71. Your questions may differ.

Muscle Dysfunction

Cardiomyopathy

Cardiomyopathy means heart muscle disease unrelated to other cardiovascular causes. It refers to a group of myocardial abnormalities with unknown causes and divergent clinical findings. Generally, cardiomyopathies fall into three categories: hypertrophic, congestive (or dilated), and restrictive (explained on pages 79 and 80). (A fourth type, obliterative cardiomyopathy, occurs in tropical areas and rarely in temperate climates.)

Assessment

Obtain a standard cardiac history and perform a physical examination. Suspect cardiomyopathy in any patient with a history of heart failure and cardiac enlargement.

Diagnostic studies. No single test diagnoses cardiomyopathies. The doctor may order an EKG, chest X-ray, echocardiogram, and possibly cardiac catheterization and nuclear studies.

Planning

Nursing priorities for a patient with cardiomyopathy depend on the disease's type and severity. As soon as your patient's condition stabilizes, teach him about his condition and help him accept it. Encourage him to comply with prescribed treatment.

Nursing diagnosis. Tailor your patient care to the type and suspected cause of cardiomyopathy. Before developing the patient's care plan, formulate a nursing diagnosis to determine his actual or potential problems, then relate them to the condition's origin or cause. Possible nursing diagnoses for the patient with cardiomyopathy include:
• knowledge deficit; related to disease
• cardiac output, alteration in (decreased); related to left ventricular failure
• noncompliance (potential for); related to inadequate health teaching
• coping, ineffective family (compromised); related to patient's disease process outcome

Continued on page 78

Sample nursing care plan: Cardiomyopathy

Nursing diagnosis	Expected outcomes
Knowledge deficit related to disease	The patient will: • show knowledge of his disease and its process • show knowledge of his care plan and treatment • show knowledge of methods used to modify his ADL, depending on how his disease progresses.

Nursing interventions	Discharge planning
• Teach the patient about his disease and its process. • Discuss the care plan and treatment rationale with the patient. Include medication teaching. • Discuss ways to modify his ADL depending on his disease state. • Give emotional support. • Allow patient to express his feelings about his condition.	• Teach the patient about his medications. • Reinforce treatment plans and the need for compliance. • Teach patient when to seek medical care. • Provide information on appropriate community service agencies.

Cardiac Problems

Muscle Dysfunction

A heart for a heart

Which patients can a human heart transplant help? Most recipients have end-stage heart disease related to congestive cardiomyopathy, or ischemic or rheumatic heart disease unresponsive to medical therapy. They're usually age 50 or younger with no history of other major diseases such as diabetes or chronic liver or lung disease.

If your patient's scheduled for transplantation, he'll undergo many preoperative tests and other forms of assessment. These tests require hospitalization, but once the workup's completed, the patient may leave the hospital until doctors find an acceptable donor.

Throughout this trying time, support and reassure the patient and his family. Prepare him psychologically for the procedure. Remember—once a donor's found, surgery must take place right away.

The donor heart must show no sign of innate disease and must be compatible with the recipient's tissue type. To assess donor heart function, the doctor may perform a cardiac catheterization. Transplantation can take place after this evaluation.

The medical team first connects the patient to a cardiopulmonary bypass machine. Next, they excise the donor and recipient hearts simultaneously. After appropriate preparation, the doctor anastomoses the donor's heart to the recipient's atrial walls, which remain in place. He then anastomoses the great vessels (aorta and pulmonary artery). Now the team weans the patient from the bypass machine and starts rewarming him.

Your postoperative care priorities include preventing infection and rejection of the new heart, and warding off cardiac complications such as dysrhythmias. Be ready to administer steroids and immunosuppressants, as ordered. Prepare your patient for regular myocardial biopsies, as indicated, to assess for early rejection signs and to guide therapy. About 50% of heart transplant recipients now survive beyond 3 years after surgery.

Cardiomyopathy—*continued*

● gas exchange, impaired; related to decreased cardiac output
● fluid volume, alteration in (excess); related to decreased pumping ability
● powerlessness; related to disease process.

You'll find a sample nursing care plan for the patient with cardiomyopathy on page 77. Remember to individualize each care plan to the needs of the patient and his family or support persons. Use this sample plan as a guide when listing expected outcomes, nursing interventions, and discharge planning.

Interventions
(See interventions described for each cardiomyopathy type.)

Evaluation
Base your evaluation of the patient with cardiomyopathy on his expected outcomes listed on his care plan. To determine if his condition's improved, ask yourself the following questions:
● Does he understand his disease and its process?
● Can he knowledgeably discuss his care plan and treatment?
● Does he know ways to modify his daily activities?
● Has he expressed his feelings about his condition?
● Does he know when to seek medical care?
● Does he know which local agencies to turn to for emotional or financial help?

The answers to these questions will help you evaluate your patient's status and the effectiveness of his care. Keep in mind that these questions stem from the sample care plan shown on page 77. Your questions may differ.

Human heart transplantation
The illustration below shows how the donor heart's attached to the recipient heart during heart transplantation.

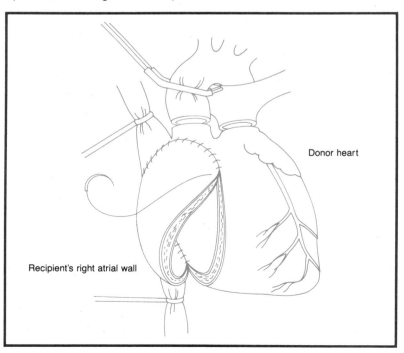

Donor heart

Recipient's right atrial wall

Muscle Dysfunction

Recent advances in cardiac disease treatment include human heart transplantation (see *A heart for a heart*, page 78, and *A mechanical boost for the failing heart*, page 73).

Cardiomyopathy types

Hypertrophic cardiomyopathy (HCM)

This may also go by the names idiopathic hypertrophic subaortic stenosis (IHSS), asymmetrical septal hypertrophy (ASH), and hypertrophic obstructive cardiomyopathy (HOCM). (However, these terms are less inclusive.) This disease, probably genetic in origin, causes pronounced ventricular hypertrophy, fibrosis, and myofibril disorganization leading to uncoordinated ventricular contraction. Ventricular hypertrophy reduces the ventricle's size, thus decreasing filling and leading to improper mitral valve function and mitral insufficiency. If septal hypertrophy also appears, left ventricular ejection may suffer.

HCM's functional effects result from ventricular stiffness and subsequent filling abnormalities. Usually, reduced muscle function occurs late, secondary to widespread muscle disease. Massive ventricular hypertrophy leads to markedly intensified systolic contractions during most of the disease's course.

An HCM patient may lack signs and symptoms until adulthood. (See the chart on page 80 for a list of signs and symptoms.)

Treatment goals for the HCM patient focus on preventing sudden death, improving ventricular filling, and relieving signs and symptoms. Drug therapy usually involves propranolol, especially if the patient has angina, dyspnea, and dysrhythmias. By decreasing heart rate and contractility, propranolol improves myocardial filling and cardiac output. In some cases, the doctor will order verapamil instead.

If angina, dysrhythmias, and congestive heart failure persist, the doctor will try to control symptoms. If medical and drug therapy fail, he may perform a septal myotomy to decrease the outflow obstruction.

Congestive (dilated) cardiomyopathy

Characterized by a large, dilated, flabby ventricular muscle, this disorder directly contrasts HCM's hypercontractile state and small ventricular chamber. Gross contractility abnormalities lead to ventricular overload, triggering CHF signs and symptoms.

Although researchers can't relate congestive cardiomyopathy to a specific cardiac cause, they've linked it to multiple MI, pregnancy and the first 6 weeks postpartum, alcoholism, chronic myocarditis, systemic hypertension, and viral illness.

A myocardial biopsy can help determine the cause of congestive cardiomyopathy. The doctor may order steroids and immunosuppressants to control any inflammation. Drug treatment resembles that for CHF: digoxin, diuretics, and vasodilators. Anticoagulants can help prevent embolism. The doctor may also order bed rest; the patient's condition will probably also limit his activity.

Continued on page 80

Unusual findings: Benign and malignant cardiac tumors

Primary cardiac tumors occur rarely, and only about 25% show cancer. But signs and symptoms of these unusual masses can confuse you.

Assess a patient with a suspected cardiac tumor for fever, cachexia (general poor health and weakness), malaise, rash, and emboli. The patient may also have chest pain, syncope, CHF, dysrhythmias, and pericarditis. Expect vague, inconclusive laboratory and physical findings.

Echocardiography (M-mode and two-dimensional) helps locate lesions and estimate their size and character. Echocardiography can also help guide the approach and technique for cardiac catheterization in a patient with a suspected lesion.

Myxomas account for about 30% to 50% of cardiac tumors. These benign masses, which may be genetically transmitted, occur most commonly in patients age 30 to 60. More myxomas occur in the left atria than the right, although biatrial and ventricular myxomas have been reported.

Signs and symptoms of myxoma mimic those of valvular disease and commonly include emboli formation.

In most cases, the doctor will surgically remove a myxoma. This usually cures the condition, although about 5% of the tumors recur. Postoperative care includes long-term follow-up evaluation with echocardiography.

Sarcomas, the second most common cardiac tumor type, occur most frequently in the right atrium. Because these cancerous tumors proliferate rapidly, most patients die within 2 years of symptom onset. Diagnosis usually starts with echocardiography. The doctor may also recommend cardiac catheterization.

Surgery may relieve sarcoma symptoms, but it rarely improves life expectancy. Chemotherapy and radiation therapy may also help relieve symptoms.

Muscle Dysfunction

Assessing cardiomyopathy

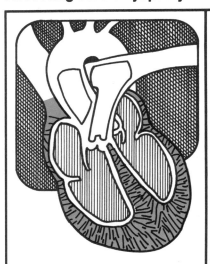

Hypertrophic cardiomyopathy

Signs and symptoms:
- exertional dyspnea
- orthopnea
- paroxysmal nocturnal dyspnea
- angina
- fatigue
- syncope
- palpitations
- ankle edema
- mild cardiomegaly
- apical systolic thrill and heave
- S_4
- systolic murmur that increases with Valsalva's maneuver

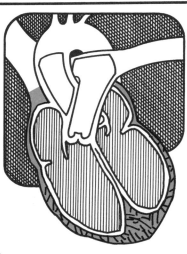

Congestive (dilated) cardiomyopathy

Signs and symptoms:
- gradual onset of signs and symptoms
- congestive heart failure (especially left-sided)
- dyspnea
- fatigue and weakness
- systemic or pulmonary emboli
- possible signs of alcoholism
- moderate-to-severe cardiomegaly
- S_3 and S_4
- atrioventricular (AV) valve regurgitation (especially mitral)

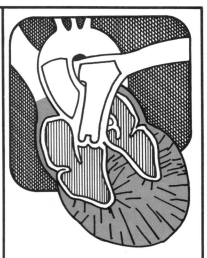

Restrictive cardiomyopathy

Signs and symptoms:
- exercise intolerance
- dyspnea
- fatigue
- right-sided congestive failure
- mild-to-moderate cardiomegaly
- S_3 and S_4
- AV valve regurgitation
- Kussmaul's sign (inspiratory venous pressure increase)

Cardiomyopathy types—*continued*

Congestive cardiomyopathy confers a poor prognosis. Half its victims die 3 to 5 years after diagnosis—usually from severe end-stage CHF.

Restrictive cardiomyopathy

The least common type, this disorder causes limited ventricular filling from myocardial cell infiltrates and fibrosis. Consequently, compliance decreases and the heart becomes stiff and hard to fill. Fibrosis causes include infiltrative diseases such as amyloidosis, endomyocardial fibrosis of tropical and humid zones, and Loffler's eosinophilic cardiomyopathy.

As the disease progresses, myocardial contractility falters, reducing cardiac output and bringing on systemic and pulmonary congestion. Restrictive cardiomyopathy may be misdiagnosed as constrictive pericarditis because it causes similar signs and symptoms.

Digoxin, diuretics, and other therapies can relieve symptoms; anticoagulants prevent emboli formation. Prognosis depends on heart failure severity as well as any embolism development. The disease usually progresses to end-stage CHF.

Inflammatory Disease: Pericarditis, Endocarditis, and Myocarditis

Rosalie A. Przykucki, who wrote this chapter, works as a staff nurse in the cardiovascular and thoracic intensive care unit at Emory University Hospital in Atlanta. She received her BSN from Emory and her MSN from Georgia State University.

Although normally a protective mechanism, inflammation can take a devastating toll on the heart. In this chapter, we'll review three types of inflammatory heart disease—pericarditis, infective endocarditis, and myocarditis.

Pericarditis

An inflammation of the pericardium, pericarditis can cause chest pain, pericardial friction rub, and serial EKG abnormalities. The most common causes include bacterial and viral infections, cardiac injury, uremia, and trauma.

Pericarditis types include:
• *constrictive pericarditis.* In this disorder, inflamed pericardial surfaces form a thick scar tissue that attracts fibrin and calcium deposits and fuses the pericardium's visceral and parietal layers. Resulting stiffening of the normally elastic pericardium prevents

Continued on page 82

The heart's outer layers: A review

Inflammatory heart disease can affect the heart wall or the surrounding pericardium. The heart wall has three layers: the inner *endocardium* (a thin layer of endothelial cells and connective tissue); the thick, muscular *myocardium* (bundles of myofibrils, or cardiac muscle fibers); and the outer *epicardium.*

The *pericardium*, a double-walled, fluid-filled sac, lubricates the beating heart and helps prevent cardiac infection by creating a barrier between the heart and other organs. In addition, the pericardium:
• holds the heart in a fixed position
• supports the great vessels, preventing them from kinking
• restrains ventricular dilation during exertion, preventing overstretching of myofibrils.

The epicardium (sometimes called the *visceral pericardium*) serves as the pericardium's inner wall; the *parietal pericardium*, a smooth, translucent membrane, serves as the pericardium's outer wall. (The parietal pericardium has an outer layer of dense, fibrous tissue called the *fibrous pericardium.*)

The cavity between the parietal pericardium and the epicardium contains 20 to 50 ml of lymphlike pericardial fluid. Pressure in the pericardial cavity, normally negative, rises intermittently during ventricular filling, forcing excess fluid into the mediastinum's lymphatic channels.

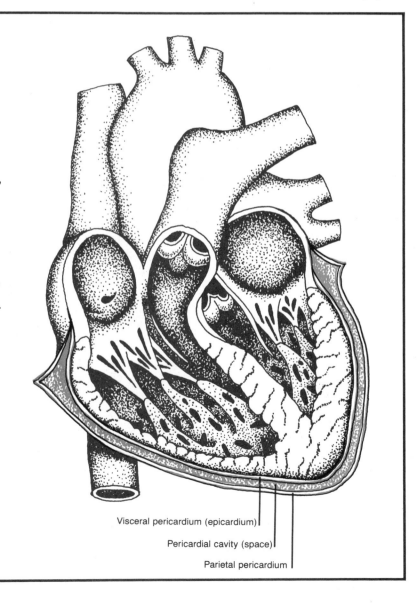

Visceral pericardium (epicardium)

Pericardial cavity (space)

Parietal pericardium

Inflammatory Diseases

Pericardial pain

Most pericardial pain originates from inflammation of the diaphragm or diaphragmatic pleura. In the pericardium itself, only the lower part of the parietal pericardium senses pain.

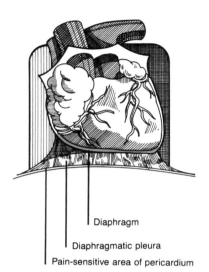

Diaphragm

Diaphragmatic pleura

Pain-sensitive area of pericardium

Pericarditis—*continued*

adequate diastolic filling. Thus, systemic venous and right atrial pressures don't drop with inspiration, and atrial filling diminishes. Eventually, stroke volume and cardiac output decrease, resulting in heart failure. Known causes of constrictive pericarditis include tuberculosis, chronic renal failure, systemic lupus erythematosus, surgery, and radiation.

• *post-myocardial infarction (post-MI) pericarditis.* Seen after a transmural MI, this pericarditis type results from fibrin deposited between the pericardial layers at the myocardial necrosis site.

• *Dressler's syndrome.* Occurring weeks to months after an MI, this disorder (probably an autoimmune disease) causes fever, pleuritis, and pericardial inflammation.

• *postcardiotomy syndrome.* This condition may develop 2 to 3 weeks after open-heart surgery. Signs and symptoms resemble those of Dressler's syndrome.

Pericarditis may be:
• acute—lasting less than 6 weeks
• subacute—lasting 6 weeks to 6 months
• chronic—lasting longer than 6 months.

Assessment

Begin with a thorough health history to identify possible pericarditis causes. Usual signs and symptoms of acute pericarditis include chest pain, pericardial friction rub, and dyspnea.

To differentiate pericarditis from MI, pinpoint the location of chest pain. Precordial or substernal chest pain of acute pericarditis, which the patient may describe as sharp and stabbing, usually localizes to the left or right shoulder, arm, elbow, and neck. Inspiration, coughing, swallowing, and trunk rotation exacerbate the pain.

When auscultating heart sounds, you may hear a grating, scratchy, or scraping sound. This indicates pericardial friction rub, caused by friction created as the pericardial and epicardial layers rub against each other. Take care to distinguish a pericardial friction rub from a murmur: murmurs radiate; pericardial friction rubs don't.

Dyspnea, frequently occurring with pericarditis, may accompany chest pain. This symptom results from compression of the bronchi or lung parenchyma by the distended pericardium. (See Chapter 1 for more information on dyspnea and heart sounds.)

Other indications of pericarditis include dysrhythmias (such as atrial fibrillation), chills, fever, and diaphoresis.

Diagnostic studies. Various tests may confirm a diagnosis of pericarditis and help determine the cause. Serial EKGs may help differentiate acute pericarditis from MI. Four EKG stages appear in pericarditis. Stage I, occurring with onset of chest pain, shows ST-segment elevation in a concave pattern. ST segments return to baseline and T waves flatten in Stage II, which usually begins within several days. In Stage III, EKG strips record T-wave inversion. The waves usually return to normal in Stage IV, weeks after the onset of acute pericarditis. A decrease in QRS voltage may also occur. These EKG changes result from myocardial inflammation

Inflammatory Diseases

and pericardial fluid or thickened pericardium, which short-circuits cardiac impulses and reduces their voltage. Other EKG abnormalities, such as atrial fibrillation or tachycardia, may occur from SA-nodal irritation.

The doctor may also order a chest X-ray and echocardiogram to identify a pericardial effusion. Cardiac enzyme tests, while not specifically indicating pericardial inflammation, may show elevated CPK-MB levels. Elevated erythrocyte sedimentation rates (ESR) and leukocytosis may also occur with pericarditis.

Planning

Your nursing care priorities for a pericarditis patient include relieving pain, preventing or reducing complications, and maintaining adequate cardiac output.

Nursing diagnoses. Potential nursing diagnoses for the pericarditis patient include:
• comfort, alteration in (pain); related to pericardial inflammation
• injury, potential for (cardiac tamponade); related to pericardial effusion
• anxiety; related to illness
• knowledge deficit; related to disease process
• noncompliance (potential for); related to inadequate health teaching
• family dynamics, alteration in; related to the disease process
• sleep pattern, disturbances in; related to pericardial pain.

For an example of a nursing care plan for a patient with pericarditis, see the box below. The sample nursing care plan shows expected outcomes, nursing interventions, and discharge planning that may be relevant to your patient. You'll want to individualize each care plan, however, to fit the needs of the patient.

Intervention

Treatment goals for the pericarditis patient include relieving pain, controlling the underlying cause, and preventing complications.

Continued on page 84

EKG changes: A comparison

Both myocardial infarction (MI) and acute pericarditis cause ST segment elevation on EKG. But, as you can see from these two illustrations, the tracings look distinctly different. Compare the ST segment and the normal T wave in the pericarditis tracing with the ST segment and the inverted T wave in the MI tracing.

Acute pericarditis

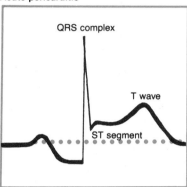

Myocardial infarction

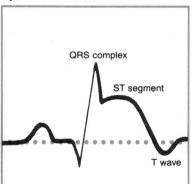

Sample nursing care plan—pericarditis

Nursing diagnosis	Expected outcomes
Comfort, alteration in (pain), related to pericardial inflammation	The patient will: • maintain an adequate level of comfort • verbalize relief • demonstrate knowledge of reason for pain medication • demonstrate knowledge of pain-control methods.
Nursing interventions • Assess for verbal and nonverbal signs and symptoms of pain. • Instruct patient to notify the nurse when pain occurs. • Check vital signs after drug administration for indications of hypotension. • After administering drugs, observe patient for relief of pain and for adverse effects of pain medication. • Discuss pain-relief methods with the patient.	**Discharge planning** • Teach patient about medication and importance of compliance. • Teach him about pericarditis and its process. • Reinforce his treatment and care plan. • Discuss pain-relief methods he can use at home. • Teach patient when to seek medical care.

Inflammatory Diseases

Understanding pericardiectomy

If your patient develops persistent or recurrent pericardial effusion (without constriction), the doctor may perform a *parietal pericardiectomy*. By removing part of the pericardium's parietal layer, this procedure permits excess pericardial fluid to drain into the pleural space. The illustration below shows the heart after surgery to remove the parietal layer, from the left phrenic nerve to the right pleural reflection, and from behind the left phrenic nerve to the pulmonary vasculature.

If constrictive pericarditis develops, the doctor may perform a *visceral pericardiectomy*. In this procedure, he removes both the parietal and endocardial (visceral) layers as necessary to free the heart from constriction.

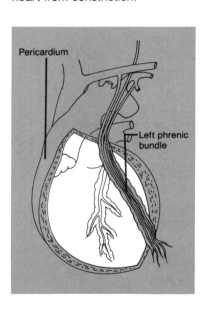

Pericarditis—*continued*

The doctor will usually treat the patient with acute pericarditis symptomatically, ordering bed rest until pain and fever disappear. Observe the patient for signs and symptoms of complications (described below). Also offer emotional support to help relieve anxiety and provide comfort measures.

To relieve pain, administer nonsteroidal anti-inflammatory agents, such as aspirin or indomethacin, as ordered. Corticosteroids, given for a short time, or left-stellate-ganglion blockade may provide additional pain relief. The doctor will usually prescribe antibiotics for bacterial pericarditis.

A patient who has recurrent, disabling pericarditis or who can't be weaned from steroids may require surgical removal of the pericardium (pericardiectomy). In most cases, however, signs and symptoms subside in 2 to 6 weeks, leaving no residual effects.

Complications

Pericardial effusion. In this disorder, excess pericardial fluid accumulates. If fluid builds up slowly, the pericardium stretches, accommodating up to 2 liters with little rise in pericardial pressure. Rapid accumulation bars pericardial stretch. The pericardium can then accommodate only 80 to 200 ml before intrapericardial pressure increases.

Large effusions can muffle heart tones and cause a paradoxical pulse, decreased cardiac output, and distended neck veins—signs of cardiac compression. If the pericardium compresses the ventricles to the point of impeding diastolic filling, cardiac output and systolic pressure decrease, signaling cardiac tamponade.

The echocardiogram most accurately and quickly identifies effusion. A chest X-ray and EKG can also help confirm pericardial effusion. Treatment of pleural effusion depends on the underlying disease and the extent of cardiac compromise.

Cardiac tamponade. This emergency occurs when fluid accumulates in the pericardial cavity, restricting diastolic ventricular filling. (See Chapter 9 for more information on cardiac tamponade.)

Chronic pericarditis. This condition can take one of four forms. *Chronic pericardial effusion* occurs after pericardial inflammation. If untreated, it can progress to constrictive pericarditis. When the pericardium becomes scarred and rigid, *constrictive pericarditis* develops. The disorder's severity depends on the rate at which pericardial scarring occurs. *Effusive-constrictive pericarditis*, caused by a thickened visceral pericardium, results in cardiac constriction with effusion between the visceral and parietal layers. *Adhesive pericarditis* involves the entire pericardium and adjoining mediastinal structures. Cardiac filling usually remains unaffected.

Evaluation

Base your evaluation of the patient's care on his expected outcomes as listed on your nursing care plan. For example, you might ask yourself these questions:

• Can the patient maintain an adequate comfort level?

• Does he understand the rationale for his treatment and medication?

Inflammatory Diseases

Why lesions localize in subacute endocarditis

What explains why vegetations localize in subacute endocarditis? This illustration suggests an answer, based on the hemodynamic theory.

In mitral insufficiency, for example, pressure gradient changes between the left atrium and the left ventricle permit rapid, jetlike regurgitant blood flow into the atrium during systole. This reduces pressure on the valve's atrial side, permitting bacteria carried by the bloodstream to adhere to the valve.

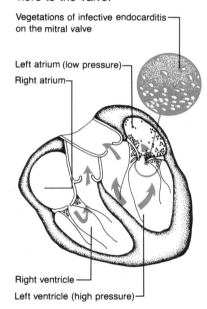

Vegetations of infective endocarditis on the mitral valve

Left atrium (low pressure)
Right atrium
Right ventricle
Left ventricle (high pressure)

• Does he know of ways to reduce pain and anxiety?

The answers to these questions will help you evaluate your patient's status and the effectiveness of his care. Keep in mind that the questions stem from the sample care plan shown on page 83. Your questions may differ.

Infective endocarditis

Formerly known as bacterial endocarditis, this microbial infection of the endothelial tissue involves the heart valves. Infective endocarditis may be acute or subacute, depending on how rapidly the disease progresses. Modern antibiotic therapy makes the previous distinction between acute and subacute forms (according to the type of invading organism) less relevant. In either form, the infecting organism adheres to the valve's endothelial surface, causing severe hemodynamic and cardiac consequences if not treated promptly. Infective endocarditis arises most frequently in patients with preexisting cardiac defects.

Mechanisms involved in infective endocarditis include:
• any bacteremia present. When organisms enter the circulation of a patient with a preexisting valvular abnormality, the abnormal valve may become infected because bacteria seed and proliferate there.
• formation of sterile platelet-fibrin thrombi. Trauma to the valvular endothelial surface, caused by turbulent blood flow or valvular disease, exposes subendothelial collagen. This substance then activates local clotting mechanisms and sterile platelet-fibrin thrombi form on the injured valve leaflets.
• any preexisting valvular damage or cardiac defects. These conditions may alter hemodynamics, causing organisms to settle outside the bloodstream and localize around the irregularities.
• the development of a high titer of agglutinating antibodies specific for the infecting organism. Circulating antibodies cause the infection to localize and spread. Platelet-fibrin thrombi provide a favorable growth environment for the organisms. Agglutinating antibodies then enhance valvular infection by causing the organisms to adhere to the thrombotic lesions.

Along with colonized bacteria clumps, these thrombi form endothelial lesions called vegetations, which tear away easily from the valvular surface. A lesion's size and shape depend on the infecting organism. Most lesions tear away easily.

Some large gram-negative vegetations may obstruct the valve orifice. In addition, erosion can cause valve leaflet rupture, while necrosis can lead to rupture of the chordae tendinae and papillary muscles.

Healing may take 2 to 3 months with antimicrobial therapy, which allows fibrin and granulated tissue to grow over the vegetations. However, scarring and calcification can lead to permanent valvular deformities.

Infective endocarditis occurs more frequently in the mitral and aortic valves than in the tricuspid and pulmonic valves. Right-sided valve infections occur more commonly in parenteral drug abusers and patients with contaminated I.V. equipment.

Continued on page 86

Inflammatory Diseases

Acute infective endocarditis:
- Staphylococcus aureus
- Hemophilus influenza
- Streptococcus pneumoniae
- Neisseria meningitidis
- Neisseria gonorrhoeae
- Gram-negative bacilli
- Fungi

Subacute infective endocarditis:
- Streptococcus viridans
- Staphylococcus epidermidis
- Nonhemolytic streptococci
- Microaerophilic streptococci
- Gram-negative bacilli
- Fungi

Infective endocarditis—*continued*

Other endocarditis forms include:

- nonbacterial thrombotic endocarditis, characterized by sterile, platelet-fibrin thrombi on cardiac valves and related to a blood-clotting problem.
- Libman-Sacks endocarditis, a nonbacterial form commonly seen in systemic lupus erythematosus patients.

A patient with known valvular heart disease may develop infective endocarditis unless given prophylactic antibiotic therapy before invasive procedures such as dental extractions and cleaning, transurethral prostate resections, bronchoscopy, or endoscopy. Microorganisms entering the circulatory system through such procedures may infect the endocardium.

How infective endocarditis can cause embolism

Dental procedures
- Extractions
- Teeth cleaning
- Denture or bridge work
- Fillings

Other invasive procedures
- Abdominal or thoracic surgery
- Tonsillectomy and other ear, nose, and throat procedures
- Bronchoscopy, endoscopy, sigmoidoscopy, and cystoscopy
- Dilatation and curettage
- I.V. therapy
- Intrauterine devices
- Cardiac pacemaker insertion

Injury or trauma
- Laceration
- Abscess
- Puncture

Inflammatory and infectious disorders
- Rashes
- Endometriosis
- Periodontal disease
- Pneumonia and other respiratory tract infections

Allow bacteria to enter the bloodstream

Bacteria collect on heart valve damaged by fibrin and platelet deposits, leading to formation of vegetations

Vegetations break loose and embolize to other organs via the bloodstream

Emboli may lodge in other organs, causing infarctions in lungs, brain, spleen, kidneys, heart

Inflammatory Diseases

Patient-teaching tip

Contact your local American Heart Association chapter for the publication *Prevention of Bacterial Endocarditis*, a valuable patient-teaching aid.

Assessment

Suspect infective endocarditis in any patient with a fever of unknown origin and a heart murmur or in a patient at high risk for developing this infection. To assess the patient's status, obtain a complete health history. The following factors can increase his endocarditis risk:

• known history of congenital or acquired cardiac disease (for example, heart murmur, congestive heart failure [CHF], rheumatic heart disease, scarlet fever, or aortic or mitral stenosis or insufficiency)
• cardiac surgery
• immunosuppression
• invasive procedures in the last year
• I.V. drug use, including hyperalimentation.

Also ask the patient to describe his symptoms, including time of onset, and find out which medications he uses and whether he has any known drug allergies.

A patient with infective endocarditis will probably have vague, nonspecific signs and symptoms of infection: malaise, fatigue, headache, cough, anorexia, and weight loss. Patients with less virulent forms may run a low-grade fever ranging from 37.2° to 38.8° C. (99° to 102° F.); patients with a fulminant disease process have high-grade fevers ranging from 39.4° to 40° C. (103° to 104° F.).

Check for signs and symptoms of CHF. A patient with infective endocarditis may not show CHF indications in the disease's early

Continued on page 88

Peripheral signs of infective endocarditis

Classic peripheral manifestations of endocarditis may stem from allergic vasculitis of the arterioles.

Retinal hemorrhages, called Roth's spots, may accompany infective endocarditis. These spots, which resemble cotton wool, may disappear suddenly.

Petechiae may cluster in the conjunctivae and other mucous membranes or around the clavicles, wrists, or ankles. Eventually, they fade to brown spots.

Splinter (subungual) hemorrhages may also occur, but they're not specific to infective endocarditis.

About 10% to 20% of endocarditis patients develop Osler's nodes on their palms or soles or on the pads of their fingers or toes. These painful, white-centered, erythematous nodes vary in size from 1 to 10 mm.

Painless, hemorrhagic Janeway lesions, which range from 1 to 5 mm in diameter, may appear on the arms, legs, palms, and soles. They become more pronounced when the patient raises his arm or leg.

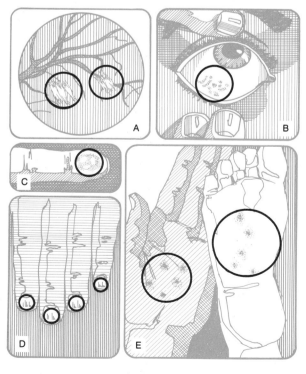

A—Roth's spots (magnified)
B—Conjunctival petechiae
C—Osler's nodes
D—Splinter hemorrhages
E—Janeway lesions

Inflammatory Diseases

Telltale signs and symptoms of infective endocarditis

Indications of infection:
• Fever, chills, diaphoresis
• Cough
• Headache
• Anorexia, weight loss
• Malaise, fatigue

Indications of cardiac injury:
• New murmur or a change in the quality or intensity of an old murmur
• Pericardial friction rub
• Congestive heart failure
• Pericarditis, myocardial infarction, or cardiac tamponade

Indications of a hypersensitivity reaction:
• Petechiae
• Splinter hemorrhages
• Osler's nodes
• Janeway lesions
• Roth's spots

Infective endocarditis—*continued*
stages. Also listen for murmurs; a patient in a later stage or one with the subacute form may have regurgitant murmurs.

Diagnostic studies. A positive blood culture can confirm infective endocarditis. Most patients also have normochromic, normocytic anemia. Leukocyte counts frequently rise in the initial stages.

Endocardial infection can cause conduction abnormalities, seen on EKG. Two-dimensional echocardiography helps visualize large valvular vegetations.

Planning
Care priorities include identifying the causative agent, relieving symptoms, and preventing complications.

Nursing diagnoses. Potential nursing diagnoses for an infective endocarditis patient include:
• injury (potential for), cardiac valve infection; related to infecting organism
• cardiac output, alteration in (decreased); related to ineffective cardiac valve functioning
• self-concept, disturbances in; related to the disease process
• anxiety, related to the disease process and hospitalization
• injury (potential for), phlebitis; related to prolonged I.V. therapy
• noncompliance (potential for); related to inadequate teaching.

For an example of a nursing care plan for the patient with infective endocarditis, see the box below. The sample nursing care plan shows expected outcomes, nursing interventions, and discharge planning that may be relevant to your patient. You'll want to individualize each care plan, however, to fit the needs of the patient.

Sample nursing care plan—infective endocarditis

Nursing diagnosis	**Expected outcomes**
Injury (potential for), cardiac valve infection, related to infecting organism	The patient will: • be free of fever, chills, and diaphoresis • maintain adequate cardiac output • demonstrate knowledge of his disease and its process • demonstrate knowledge of the reason/rationale for his treatment • demonstrate knowledge of procedures requiring prophylactic antibiotics.
Nursing interventions • Assess vital signs, watching for signs of fever and decreased cardiac output. • After giving antipyretics and antibiotics, monitor patient for adverse reactions and adequate response. • Encourage fluid intake. • Provide cooling measures, such as ice packs to the neck, axilla, or groin, if indicated. • Discuss the disease and its process with the patient. • Discuss the treatment and care plan with the patient.	**Discharge planning** • Teach patient how to take his temperature and how to recognize signs and symptoms of infection. • Reinforce care plan and the need for compliance with treatment and follow-up care. • Teach patient about his medications. • Teach him when to seek medical care. • Advise him to alert doctor when undergoing any invasive procedure.

Inflammatory Diseases

Intervention

Treatment goals include eradicating the infecting organism and preventing complications and relapse.

Antimicrobial therapy depends on the infecting microorganism. Early administration (usually I.V.) improves recovery. If necessary, the doctor will surgically replace the infected valve. (See Chapter 7 for information on valve replacement.)

To help prevent complications, assess the patient thoroughly and regularly.

To help stabilize the patient's condition, limit his activities and make sure he gets adequate rest. As his condition improves, gradually schedule new activities. Also, teach the patient and his family about the disease, including its process and prevention of recurrences.

Complications

Endocardial vegetations can lead to ventricular septal defects, abscesses, pericarditis, MI, and CHF (a common cause of death in patients with infective endocarditis).

If vegetative lesions tear apart from the endocardial surfaces, ce-

Continued on page 90

Suggested treatment for infective endocarditis caused by gram-positive cocci

Organism	Antibiotic regimen	Duration (weeks)
Alpha-hemolytic (viridans) streptococci, *Streptococcus bovis*	• Penicillin G 2 million units every 6 h I.V. *plus* streptomycin 10 mg/kg every 12 h I.M., or	2
	• Penicillin G 2 million units every 6 h I.V. *plus* streptomycin 10 mg/kg every 12 h I.M. (for first 2 weeks only), or	4
	• Penicillin G 4 million units every 6 h I.V., or	4
	• Cefazolin 2 g every 6 h I.V., or	4
	• Vancomycin 15 mg/kg every 12 h I.V.	4
Group A streptococci, *Streptococcus pneumoniae*	• Penicillin G 3 million units every 6 h I.V., or	2 to 4
	• Cefazolin 2 g every 6 h I.V.	2 to 4
Streptococcus fecalis, other penicillin-resistant streptococci	• Ampicillin 2 g every 4 h I.V. *plus* gentamicin 1.5 mg/kg every 8 h I.V., or	4 to 6
	• Vancomycin 15 mg/kg every 12 h I.V. *plus* streptomycin 15 mg/kg every 12 h I.M.	4 to 6
Staphylococcus aureus	• Nafcillin 2 g every 4 h I.V., or	4 or longer
	• Nafcillin as above *plus* gentamicin 1.5 mg/kg every 8 h I.V. for the first 5 days, or	4 or longer
	• Cephalothin 2 g every 4 h I.V., or	4 or longer
	• Vancomycin 500 mg every 6 h I.V.	4 or longer

Source: J. Willis Hurst, *The Heart* (New York: McGraw-Hill Co., 1982)

Inflammatory Diseases

Rheumatic fever: Another inflammatory heart disease

Also known as rheumatic heart disease, rheumatic fever can cause chronic heart problems stemming from an acute inflammatory reaction to a Group A betahemolytic streptococcal pharyngeal infection. The affected tissue develops small, necrotic areas (Aschoff bodies) that leave scar tissue after they heal. If scarred, valves become fibrous and incompetent. Cardiac complications, such as pericarditis, endocarditis, or myocarditis, may appear years after the streptococcal infection. (See Chapter 7 for more information on valvular disease.)

Infective endocarditis—*continued*

rebral, renal, or splenic emboli can develop. These complications may arise at any point—even weeks or months after treatment.

Evaluation

Base your evaluation on the expected outcomes listed on your nursing care plan. For example, you might ask yourself the following questions:
- Does the patient have a fever, chills, diaphoresis, or other signs of infection?
- Does he have adequate cardiac output?
- Does he understand the disease process and his treatment plan?

The answers to these questions will help you evaluate your patient's status and the effectiveness of his care. Keep in mind that these questions stem from the sample care plan on page 88. Your questions may differ.

Myocarditis

This inflammation of the myocardium may result from a viral, bacterial, or autoimmune disease and less commonly from exposure to radiation, chemotherapy, or other drugs and chemicals. Myocarditis sometimes leads to acute congestive cardiomyopathy.

Myocardial damage comes about through one of three mechanisms:
- invasion by the causative agent
- myocardial toxin production
- autoimmunity.

The disease's course depends on the size, number, and location of lesions. The disease can affect a patient of any age. Some patients

How viral myocarditis develops

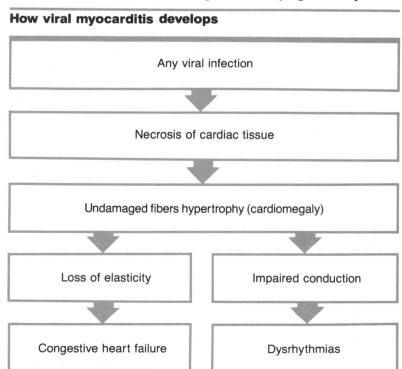

Any viral infection

↓

Necrosis of cardiac tissue

↓

Undamaged fibers hypertrophy (cardiomegaly)

↓

Loss of elasticity → Congestive heart failure

Impaired conduction → Dysrhythmias

Inflammatory Diseases

with the acute form respond successfully to treatment, leaving no residual effects. Others may progress to cardiomyopathy or die.

Assessment
Begin by obtaining a complete health history. Ask the patient if he's recently had radiation therapy, chemotherapy, or a viral or bacterial infection. Ask which, if any, medications he uses, and note the frequency and duration of use. Also ask about known drug allergies.

Expect vague, varied signs and symptoms. The patient may complain of fatigue, dyspnea, palpitations, or pericardial discomfort. Check for an elevated temperature. Tachycardia may accompany a fever, but usually to an extent disproportionate to the degree of elevation.

Diagnostic studies. The patient's systemic symptoms usually help diagnose myocarditis. An increase in complement-fixation, virus-neutralizing antibody, or hemagglutination-inhibition titers may also aid diagnosis of some forms.

The patient's EKG may show a nonspecific abnormality such as supraventricular tachycardia; ventricular dysrhythmias; low-voltage QRS complexes (secondary to myocardial edema); atrioventricular conduction defects (secondary to AV node or bundle-branch inflammation); ST-segment abnormalities; or T-wave abnormalities.

Planning
Care priorities for the myocarditis patient include identifying the causative agent, relieving symptoms, preventing complications, and providing supportive care.

Because myocarditis progresses slowly, the patient will probably require long-term hospitalization. Gradually add activities to his schedule, such as those used in cardiac rehabilitation programs. After the patient's condition stabilizes, plan rest periods and a gradual resumption of normal activities.

Nursing diagnoses. Possible nursing diagnoses for the myocarditis patient include:
- self-concept, disturbances in; related to the disease process
- coping, ineffective family; related to the disease process
- skin integrity, impairment of (potential); related to bed rest
- knowledge deficit, related to the disease
- noncompliance (potential for), related to inadequate teaching.

For an example of a nursing care plan for the myocarditis patient, see the box on page 92. The sample nursing care plan shows expected outcomes, nursing interventions, and discharge planning that may be relevant to your patient. You'll want to individualize each care plan, however, to fit the needs of the patient.

Intervention
Treatment goals include controlling the inflammation, reducing the heart's work load, and preventing complications.

If the inflammation's bacterial, administer antibiotics, as ordered. Viral causes, such as Coxsackie B and echovirus, can lead to temporary or permanent changes in myocardial cell structure. The Coxsackie B virus proves particularly virulent in infants and children, causing respiratory distress, CHF, and circulatory collapse.

Continued on page 92

Inflammatory Diseases

Myocarditis—*continued*

Sample nursing care plan—myocarditis

Nursing diagnosis	Expected outcomes
Self-concept, disturbances in, related to disease process	The patient will: • help determine his treatment plan • perform daily hygiene with minimal assistance • interact with family members and nursing staff • participate in his scheduled exercise activities.
Nursing interventions • Discuss disease and its process with patient. • Allow patient to verbalize feelings about his disease. • Plan a daily schedule of activities with the patient. Post schedule in a visible place. • Provide periods of uninterrupted rest for the patient. • Encourage family members or support persons to assist in patient's care plan.	**Discharge planning** • Teach patient about disease process. • Reinforce treatment plan and need for compliance. • Encourage patient to assume responsibility for his care. • Refer him to appropriate community agencies for additional support. • Teach him when to seek medical attention. • Help him plan ways to modify his activities of daily living.

Adults usually recover without residual symptoms. The doctor will probably order symptomatic treatment for viral inflammations.

To reduce the heart's work load, decrease residual myocardial damage, and promote healing, place the patient on bed rest and restrict physical activity. Administer oxygen, as ordered, to decrease tissue oxygen demands. As ordered, give antipyretic agents to control fever, if present. (Fever increases the heart's work load.) Make sure the patient receives adequate nutrition.

If the patient has CHF, restrict fluids and sodium intake. The doctor may order digoxin to control supraventricular tachycardia and improve myocardial contractility.

Complications

Stay alert for indications of CHF, dysrhythmias, heart block, and pulmonary or systemic emboli. Myocarditis increases a patient's sensitivity to diuretics and digitalis, so assess frequently for signs of digitalis toxicity.

Evaluation

Base your evaluation of the patient on his expected outcomes as listed on your nursing care plan. For example, you might ask yourself the following questions:
• Does the patient understand his condition and its process?
• Does he understand his treatment plan?
• Does he take responsibility for self-care?
• Does he know when to seek medical advice?
• Does he know of appropriate community referral agencies?
• Does he know how to modify his activities of daily living (ADL) to suit his condition?

The answers to these questions will help you evaluate your patient's condition and the effectiveness of his care. Keep in mind that these questions stem from the sample care plan above. Your questions may differ.

Valvular Heart Disease: Disruption of the Heart's Blood Flow

Theresa M. Boley, who wrote this chapter, is a clinical research associate in thoracic surgery at the University of Missouri in Columbia. A nursing graduate of Trenton (Mo.) Junior College, she's currently pursuing her BSN at the University of Missouri.

No matter what the underlying cause, a valvular heart disease prevents efficient blood flow through the heart. Depending on the disorder's severity and the number of valves involved, a patient with valvular disease may face heart failure, dysrhythmias, and other life-threatening complications.

The two main types of valvular disease include *stenosis* (valvular tissue thickening that narrows the valvular opening) and *insufficiency* (valvular incompetence, that prevents complete valve closure). Stenosis limits blood flow through the heart, increasing afterload (*pressure* overload). Valvular insufficiency (also called regurgitation) permits blood backflow, which increases preload (*volume* overload). Thus, both stenosis and insufficiency increase the heart's work load.

A third valvular disorder, *mitral valve prolapse*, occurs when valve leaflets protrude into the left atrium during systole. Although usually benign, this condition may lead to mitral insufficiency in a few patients.

Continued on page 94

How heart valves control blood flow

The heart's four valves, which consist of endothelium covered by fibrous tissue, regulate blood flow through the heart by opening and closing in response to pressure changes in the heart chambers.

The atrioventricular (AV) valves control blood flow from the atria into the ventricles. The *tricuspid valve*, which connects the right atrium to the right ventricle, consists of three cusps (endothelial flaps). The *mitral*, or *bicuspid, valve* has two cusps and connects the left atrium to the left ventricle.

When atrial pressure exceeds ventricular pressure, the AV valves open and blood flows into the ventricles. During systole, rising ventricular pressure forces the valves closed. The chordae tendineae also help keep the valves closed.

The semilunar valves (with their three half-moon–shaped cusps) control blood outflow from the ventricles. When right ventricular pressure exceeds pulmonary artery pressure, the *pulmonic valve* opens and allows blood to flow to the lungs. Similarly, when left ventricular pressure exceeds aortic pressure, the *aortic valve* opens and blood enters the systemic circulation.

The illustration, *right*, shows how the heart's valves look during diastole, viewed from the base of the heart with the atria removed. Note the closed semilunar valves and the open AV valves.

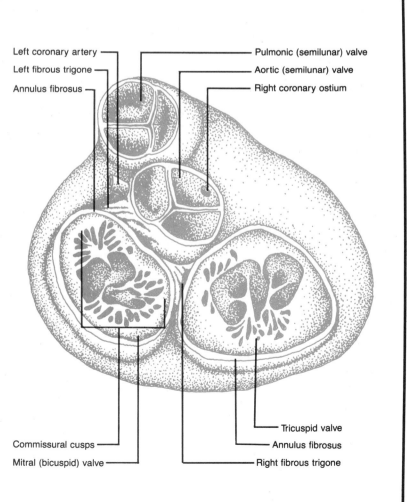

Left coronary artery
Left fibrous trigone
Annulus fibrosus

Pulmonic (semilunar) valve
Aortic (semilunar) valve
Right coronary ostium

Commissural cusps
Mitral (bicuspid) valve

Tricuspid valve
Annulus fibrosus
Right fibrous trigone

Valvular Heart Disease

LAP waveform: Picturing mitral insufficiency

If your patient has a left atrial catheter in place, you can identify mitral insufficiency by observing the waveform tracing during left atrial pressure (LAP) monitoring. On the waveform shown below, the heightened *v* wave indicates blood regurgitation through the mitral valve during ventricular contraction. ·

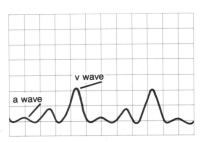

Normal waveform

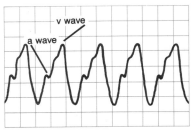

Waveform of mitral insufficiency

Continued

Assessment

As always, begin by taking a thorough patient history. Be sure to ask him about his personal and family history of heart disease and rheumatic fever. Also ask about invasive procedures. And don't overlook the obvious—ask him how he feels. A tendency to become fatigued easily occurs with most valvular disorders.

Keep in mind that a patient can have more than one valvular disease (multivalvular disease). For example, he may have both aortic insufficiency and mitral stenosis.

For assessment guidelines specific to each valvular disorder, read pages 96 to 101. To review diagnostic tests for valvular disorders, see the table on page 95.

Planning

Once the doctor confirms a diagnosis of valvular disease, your care

Identifying murmurs in valvular heart disease

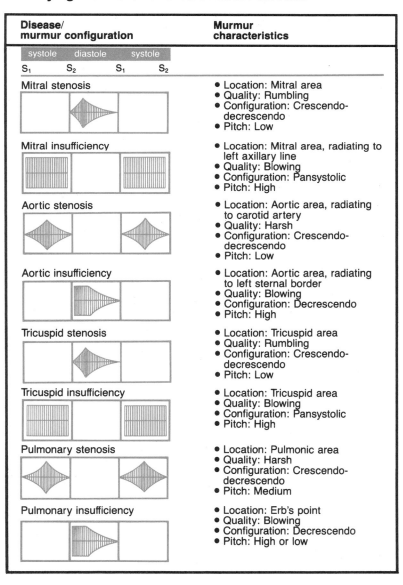

Disease/ murmur configuration	Murmur characteristics
Mitral stenosis	• Location: Mitral area • Quality: Rumbling • Configuration: Crescendo-decrescendo • Pitch: Low
Mitral insufficiency	• Location: Mitral area, radiating to left axillary line • Quality: Blowing • Configuration: Pansystolic • Pitch: High
Aortic stenosis	• Location: Aortic area, radiating to carotid artery • Quality: Harsh • Configuration: Crescendo-decrescendo • Pitch: Low
Aortic insufficiency	• Location: Aortic area, radiating to left sternal border • Quality: Blowing • Configuration: Decrescendo • Pitch: High
Tricuspid stenosis	• Location: Tricuspid area • Quality: Rumbling • Configuration: Crescendo-decrescendo • Pitch: Low
Tricuspid insufficiency	• Location: Tricuspid area • Quality: Blowing • Configuration: Pansystolic • Pitch: High
Pulmonary stenosis	• Location: Pulmonic area • Quality: Harsh • Configuration: Crescendo-decrescendo • Pitch: Medium
Pulmonary insufficiency	• Location: Erb's point • Quality: Blowing • Configuration: Decrescendo • Pitch: High or low

Valvular Heart Disease

Possible diagnostic findings in valvular disease

Use the table below as a guide to diagnostic test findings that may indicate valvular disease. (*Note:* The doctor may use cardiac catheterization as a diagnostic adjunct to determine the disease's extent.)

Mitral stenosis
• *X-ray:* Calcification, left atrial enlargement
• *EKG:* Atrial fibrillation
• *Echocardiogram:* Abnormal valve movement

Mitral insufficiency
• *X-ray:* Cardiac enlargement
• *EKG:* Abnormal P wave, indicating left atrial enlargement
• *Echocardiogram:* Left atrial and ventricular enlargement, changes in valve leaflets

Mitral valve prolapse
• *X-ray:* Normal
• *EKG:* Normal or show ST and T wave changes, supraventricular dysrhythmias, or conduction disturbances
• *Echocardiogram:* Abnormal movement of mitral valve leaflet

Aortic stenosis
• *X-ray:* Normal size heart or left ventricular enlargement and pulmonary congestion (in late stages)
• *EKG:* Regular rhythm, large S waves in right precordial leads; large R waves in left precordial leads, with ST segment depression and inverted T waves
• *Echocardiogram:* Left ventricular enlargement; thickening, calcification, and decreased mobility of valve cusps

Aortic insufficiency
• *X-ray:* Left ventricular enlargement, congested pulmonary vasculature
• *EKG:* Increased QRS amplitude and ST-T wave depression (if patient has normal sinus rhythm), indicating left ventricular enlargement
• *Echocardiogram:* Abnormal movement (fluttering) of mitral valve, cardiac enlargement

Tricuspid stenosis
• *X-ray:* Right atrial enlargement, displacement of right heart border to right
• *EKG:* Peaked P waves, indicating right artrial enlargement
• *Echocardiogram:* Thickened, scarred valve

Tricuspid insufficiency
• *X-ray:* Right heart enlargement
• *EKG:* Peaked P waves, showing axis deviation from right heart enlargement
• *Echocardiogram:* Abnormal movement

Pulmonary stenosis
• *X-ray:* Decreased pulmonary vascular markings, right ventricular enlargement
• *EKG:* Normal or show right axis deviation and ventricular enlargement
• *Echocardiogram:* Right ventricular enlargement

Pulmonary insufficiency
• *X-ray:* Right ventricular enlargement
• *EKG:* Normal or show right axis deviation and ventricular enlargement
• *Echocardiogram:* Right ventricular enlargement

priorities include maintaining adequate cardiac output, controlling pain, preventing complications (such as dysrhythmias, infection, and congestive heart failure), and patient teaching.

Teaching may be your biggest challenge. If the patient lacks symptoms at the time of diagnosis, help him understand why he needs continuous follow-up assessment and care to prevent (or slow) deterioration in his condition. Explain why he needs prophylactic antibiotic therapy before any surgical or dental procedures. If appropriate, discuss the possibility of valve repair or replacement surgery with him.

Nursing diagnoses. Your nursing diagnoses may include some or all of the following:
• knowledge deficit; related to valve surgery
• tissue perfusion, alteration in; related to valve abnormality
• activity intolerance; related to decreased cardiac output
• cardiac output, alteration in (decreased); related to valvular disease
• knowledge deficit; related to disease process
• injury (embolus), potential for; related to valvular disease.

The sample nursing care plan (below) for the patient with a valvular heart disease lists expected outcomes, nursing interventions, and discharge planning for one of the nursing diagnoses listed above. You'll want to individualize each care plan, however, to fit the needs of the patient and his family.

Intervention

For the patient with a valvular disease, nursing and medical interventions focus on preventing the disease from worsening, minimizing the risk of complications, and patient education. If the patient's condition can't be managed medically, however, the doctor may recommend another option: surgery either to repair the defective valve or to replace it. Repair procedures include:
• *valvuloplasty* to repair the valve and suture torn leaflets
• *annuloplasty* to tighten and suture the malfunctioning valve annulus (ring)

Continued on page 96

Sample nursing care plan—valvular disease

Nursing diagnosis Knowledge deficit; related to valvular surgery (valve replacement)	**Expected outcomes** The patient will: • show knowledge of his disease and its process • show knowledge of the type of surgery he's scheduled for (valve replacement) • show knowledge of preoperative and postoperative care and management • participate in his care planning and implementation.
Nursing interventions • Teach the patient about the type of surgery he's scheduled for (valve replacement) and the preoperative and postoperative care involved. • Reinforce teaching during patient care. • Encourage the patient to express his feelings about surgery. • Teach him about his disease and how it may progress.	**Discharge planning** • Teach the patient when to seek medical care. • Reinforce the treatment plan and need for compliance with therapy (such as anticoagulants). • Discuss plans for follow-up care.

Valvular Heart Disease

Continued

• *commissurotomy or valvotomy*, mechanical dilation of the valve's commissures to enlarge the valve opening.

In some cases, the doctor may remove the valve and replace it with a prosthetic device. He can choose from two prosthetic valve types. *Mechanical* prosthetic valves, while durable, may cause thrombo-embolism or fail mechanically. To minimize embolism risk, the patient must undergo anticoagulant therapy for the rest of his life.

Bioprosthetic valves (human or animal heart valves) don't require prolonged anticoagulant therapy; however, they're less durable than mechanical valves and may calcify (especially in patients with renal disease).

At best, a prosthetic valve relieves symptoms, but won't cure the disease. In general, the longer the patient had symptoms before surgery, the less likely that a prosthetic valve will give full relief.

In addition to the inherent risks of open-heart surgery, complications of valve replacement surgery include thromboembolism, hemolysis and hemolytic anemia, prosthetic valve dysfunction, and prosthetic valve endocarditis.

When your patient's scheduled for surgery, provide thorough patient teaching and preoperative care, according to hospital protocol. To guard against infective endocarditis, administer prophylactic antibiotic therapy, as ordered. After valve replacement surgery, administer anticoagulant therapy to maintain prothrombin time at 1½ to 2 times the patient's preoperative measurement, as ordered.

Evaluation

Base your evaluation on the patient's expected outcomes listed on your nursing care plan. To determine whether his condition's improved, ask yourself the following questions:
• Does the patient know about his disease and how it may progress?
• Did he receive adequate preoperative and postoperative teaching?
• Does he understand his treatment plan?
• Does he help plan and implement his care?

The answers to these questions will help you evaluate your patient's status and the effectiveness of his care. Keep in mind that these questions stem from the care plan shown on page 95. Your questions may differ.

Valvular disease types

Valvular disorders can affect any of the heart's four valves. Let's take a closer look, starting with the valves on the left side.

Left-sided valve disease
Mitral stenosis. This thickening and contracture of the valve cusps progressively obstructs blood flow. The chordae tendineae sometimes shorten and fuse together, and valve leaflets may calcify, becoming rigid and immobile. The most common cause? Rheumatic fever, although stenosis may also accompany congenital disorders.

The patient's signs and symptoms reflect pulmonary congestion, reduced cardiac output, and right ventricular failure. Because the stenotic mitral valve inhibits blood flow into the left ventricle, blood

Prosthetic heart valves: Some examples

When choosing among prosthetic valves, the doctor weighs such factors as design, durability, and hemodynamic qualities. He also considers patient compliance for this reason: mechanical prostheses encourage thrombus formation, so the patient must undergo lifelong anticoagulant therapy and regular prothrombin time testing. For a patient unlikely to comply, the doctor may select a bioprosthesis instead because it doesn't require long-term anticoagulant therapy.

The following illustrations show several available prosthetic types.

Starr-Edwards ball cage mechanical valve

The *ball cage* mechanical valve, (shown above), while durable, won't be used for tricuspid valve replacement because it's too large for the right ventricle.

Bjork-Shiley tilting disk mechanical valve

Because of its flat design, the *tilting disk* (shown above) mechanical valve requires less space than the ball cage valve.

St. Jude's bileaflet mechanical valve

Among mechanical valve types, the *bileaflet* valve (shown above) creates the least resistance to blood flow, making it hemodynamically efficient.

Ionescu-Shiley porcine bioprosthesis

Carpentier-Edwards porcine bioprosthesis

The two *porcine bioprostheses* (shown above) require anticoagulant therapy for only about 3 months after implantation. Although less durable than mechanical prostheses, they usually don't cause thrombus formation after healing's complete.

Valvular Heart Disease

backs up in the pulmonary vasculature (causing pulmonary hypertension) and eventually, the right ventricle (causing it to enlarge and fail). When right ventricular failure develops, the patient experiences peripheral edema, hepatomegaly, and ascites. He may also have episodes of angina or syncope associated with reduced cardiac output and systemic hypotension.

To assess mitral stenosis, palpate the patient's carotid artery. Although the rhythm may be normal, you'll probably note reduced amplitude, reflecting diminished cardiac output. Next, palpate his abdomen for tenderness, ascites, and hepatomegaly. Assess his arms and legs for edema, especially pedal and pretibial edema. Next, auscultate for a diastolic rumble with an opening snap. Also listen for a prolonged first heart sound. (For more on heart murmurs, see the chart on page 94.)

Note whether the patient's dyspneic, a sign of pulmonary congestion. Also assess for hemoptysis and orthopnea. Ask the patient if he's had episodes of chest pain, a possible result of hypoxia from reduced cardiac output.

As a rule, an asymptomatic patient needs no therapy. But if atrial fibrillation or congestive heart failure develops, the doctor will try to manage symptoms conservatively by ordering digitalis, diuretics, and a low-sodium diet. He'll consider surgery if:
• congestive heart failure resists medical management
• atrial fibrillation resists medical management, thereby increasing the risk of emboli and such complications as stroke or myocardial infarction
• the heart enlarges significantly (even if the patient's asymptomatic).

To enlarge the valve and relieve symptoms, the doctor may perform a commissurotomy, usually as an open-heart procedure.

A closed procedure, now rarely done, avoids putting the patient on a cardiopulmonary bypass machine. However, unlike the open procedure, the closed procedure doesn't allow the doctor to see the valve he's treating. When performing a closed procedure, the doctor makes a stab wound in the atrium. Then he places his finger through the atrium into the mitral valve and separates the leaflets.

Continued on page 98

Mitral insufficiency: The route to right ventricular failure	**Mitral stenosis: Progressive blood flow obstruction**
Systolic regurgitation through mitral valve ▼	Stenotic mitral valve leads to elevated left atrial pressure ▼
Left atrial dilation ▼	Left atrial dilation ▼
Left ventricular hypertrophy ▼	Fixed left-sided heart output ▼
Left ventricular failure ▼	Dyspnea, elevated pulmonary venous pressure, pulmonary edema or congestion, cyanosis ▼
Elevated pulmonary venous pressure ▼	Right ventricular and atrial enlargement ▼
Pulmonary edema or dyspnea, pulmonary congestion ▼	Right ventricular failure ▼
Elevated pulmonary artery pressure ▼	Neck vein distention, hepatomegaly ▼
Slight right ventricular enlargement ▼	Ascites ▼
Possible right ventricular failure with ascites and peripheral edema	Peripheral edema

Valvular Heart Disease

Valvular disease types—*continued*

The doctor probably won't do a commissurotomy if the patient has mitral insufficiency in addition to stenosis. If the valve's rigid, a commissurotomy won't correct stenosis. And if the valve's calcified, the procedure could dislodge an embolus.

Mitral insufficiency. This may result from a congenital defect or arise after disease (especially rheumatic fever) or trauma. When caused by rheumatic fever, mitral insufficiency usually accompanies mitral stenosis. Myxomatous degeneration, another possible cause, makes the valve gelatinous, soft, and floppy. Valve calcification and stretching of the mitral valve's annulus (which may occur secondary to ventricular dilation) can also cause insufficiency. Other possible causes include rupture of the papillary muscle or chordae tendineae and infective endocarditis.

Like mitral stenosis, mitral insufficiency causes pulmonary hypertension and right heart failure. Initially, the patient will probably have dyspnea and fatigue.

When assessing the patient, look for signs of heart failure; for example, peripheral edema, hepatomegaly, ascites, and jugular vein distention. Ask him if he tires easily or has episodes of dizziness or fainting. Also auscultate for abnormal heart sounds.

Medical management resembles that for mitral stenosis. If conservative measures fail, the doctor may repair the defective valve with annuloplasty or implant a prosthetic valve.

Mitral valve prolapse. Also called floppy mitral valve syndrome, Barlow's syndrome, or billowing mitral valve, this disorder ranks as the most common valvular abnormality. Possible causes include myxomatous degeneration, papillary muscle ischemia, mitral valve ring dysfunction, rheumatic fever (especially in young people), and ischemic heart disease (primarily in adults).

A patient with mitral valve prolapse may not have signs and symptoms. If the condition progresses, however, he may complain of fatigue, palpitations, chest pain, and syncope. He may also develop supraventricular or ventricular dysrhythmias or chordae tendineae rupture. In a few patients, the condition progresses to severe mitral insufficiency.

Assess the patient for pectus excavatum (funnel chest) or scoliosis. These abnormalities may signify a connective tissue disorder (such as Marfan's syndrome), which may cause mitral valve prolapse. Also auscultate for a high-frequency click, which you may hear at various points in the cardiac cycle. You may also hear a pansystolic or late systolic murmur.

If supraventricular tachycardia or premature ventricular contractions develop, the doctor may order propranolol. But if mitral insufficiency arises, he may replace the valve.

Aortic stenosis. This may result from fibrosis or calcification of the aortic valve, rheumatic fever, or syphilis. When caused by rheumatic fever, aortic stenosis almost always accompanies mitral valve disease.

A patient with aortic stenosis may experience angina—even if he's

Valvular Heart Disease

free of coronary artery disease. Because stenosis prevents the left ventricle from emptying completely during systole, blood pressure builds in the ventricle, possibly causing the ventricle's wall to become ischemic. Meanwhile, the heart's oxygen needs increase as it labors to pump blood through the stenotic valve, thereby worsening the ischemia and causing pain.

A patient with aortic stenosis may also complain of syncope. Here's why: Increased blood pressure inside the left ventricle stimulates baroreceptors, which respond by causing peripheral vasodilation. In combination with decreased cardiac output, peripheral vasodilation leads to hypotension, making the patient susceptible to dizziness and syncope.

He's also likely to develop left heart failure and pulmonary hypertension because the heart can't completely empty the left ventricle during systole. Look for this telltale clue: delayed carotid artery pulsation. Also assess for dyspnea and moist lung sounds (crackles), indicating pulmonary edema.

As the compromised left ventricle struggles to pump against rising pressure, it dilates and shifts position. Thus, you may note that the point of maximal impulse (PMI) has shifted laterally.

Because the stenotic aortic valve can't close normally, you won't hear the aortic component of the second heart sound. However, you'll probably hear a murmur.

Although uncommon, right heart failure may develop if the patient's condition worsens. Assess him for such characteristic signs and symptoms as peripheral edema, abdominal tenderness, hepatomegaly, and ascites.

An asymptomatic patient needs no treatment. But once he begins to experience symptoms (for example, angina or syncope), the doctor will most likely perform surgery to replace the valve. Risks associated with aortic valve replacement include embolism (from plaque dislodgment during removal of a calcified valve) and damage to the heart's conduction system. Without surgery, the patient will probably die within 3 years.

Continued on page 100

Aortic insufficiency: When blood flows backward

Diastolic regurgitation through aortic valve
▼
Left ventricular failure
▼
Left ventricular hypertrophy
▼
Left ventricular dilation
▼
Chest pain, syncope
▼
Pulmonary congestion
▼
Dyspnea, pulmonary edema
▼
Right ventricular failure

Aortic stenosis: From narrowed valve to right ventricular failure

Stenotic aortic valve leads to elevated left ventricular systolic pressure
▼
Left ventricular hypertrophy
▼
Left ventricular dilation
▼
Left ventricular failure
▼
Chest pain, syncope
▼
Elevated left atrial pressure
▼
Pulmonary congestion
▼
Dyspnea, pulmonary edema
▼
Right ventricular failure

Valvular Heart Disease

Valvular disease types—*continued*

Aortic insufficiency. This disorder has many possible causes, including rheumatic fever, infective endocarditis, dissecting aortic aneurysm, and syphilis. In a patient with severe prolonged hypertension, aortic root dilation may cause aortic insufficiency. Possible congenital causes include tetralogy of Fallot, ventricular septal defect, and coarctation of the aorta.

If your patient has early-stage aortic insufficiency, his heart may beat with unusual force, possibly causing visible carotid pulsations. As his condition progresses, he'll have dyspnea on exertion and other indications of left heart failure. Eventually, he may also develop right heart failure.

Assess for a widened pulse pressure and auscultate for a diminished second heart sound (S_2)—both resulting from valvular incompetence. Expect a normal first heart sound (S_1).

Note: Because of its sudden onset, acute insufficiency may not be accompanied by all the signs and symptoms of chronic insufficiency. However, the patient will usually experience dyspnea, indicating rapidly developing pulmonary edema.

If signs and symptoms develop, the doctor tries to manage them medically (for example, with digitalis and diuretics). If medical management fails or if the disorder results from trauma or a dissecting aorta, the patient may require surgery.

Right-sided valve disease

Tricuspid stenosis. This may accompany mitral valve disease caused by rheumatic fever. Less commonly, it develops after infective endocarditis.

The patient may complain that he's easily fatigued, reflecting low cardiac output. He may also report a fluttering sensation in his neck: giant A waves of the jugular veins, characteristic of tricuspid stenosis. These result from obstructed venous return. Also look for cyanosis, suggesting insufficient blood flow to the lungs, and signs of right heart failure.

Tricuspid stenosis: How edema develops	Tricuspid insufficiency: How it progresses
Stenotic tricuspid valve leads to elevated right atrial pressure	Systolic regurgitation through tricuspid valve
▼	▼
Right atrial dilation	Right atrial dilation
▼	▼
Systemic venous congestion	Right ventricular dilation
▼	▼
Neck vein distention	Right ventricular failure
▼	▼
Hepatomegaly, jaundice, cirrhosis	Pulmonary congestion, pleural effusion
▼	▼
Ascites	Neck vein distention
▼	▼
Peripheral edema	Hepatomegaly
	▼
	Ascites
	▼
	Edema

Valvular Heart Disease

When auscultating the heart, listen for a murmur that's shorter, softer, and more highly pitched than the murmur associated with mitral stenosis. The opening snap will be more intense with inspiration.

To reduce the right heart's work load, the doctor will order a low-sodium diet and possibly a diuretic to reduce venous return. Because tricuspid stenosis rarely occurs alone, however, he may recommend surgery before another valve malfunctions. If possible, he'll perform a commissurotomy. However, a calcified, immobile valve requires replacement—probably with a bioprosthetic valve because a mechanical valve usually won't fit into the right ventricular space.

Tricuspid insufficiency. This defect may accompany right ventricular dilation secondary to pulmonary hypertension, right ventricular infarction, or right ventricular failure. Tricuspid insufficiency also occurs with tricuspid stenosis from rheumatic fever. Other possible causes include infective endocarditis, papillary muscle dysfunction, and myxomatous degeneration.

Look for signs and symptoms of right heart failure. Also assess for nausea, vomiting, and anorexia from chronic vascular congestion of the gastrointestinal tract; seesaw chest movement during respiration, indicating enlargement of the heart's right side; peripheral edema and ascites; hepatomegaly; and atrial fibrillation.

The disorder may resolve after treatment of the underlying disease. If tricuspid insufficiency develops during end-stage right ventricular failure, the doctor probably won't perform surgery. Instead, he'll order aggressive medical therapy. But he'll probably perform bioprosthetic valve replacement for chronic insufficiency associated with myxomatous degeneration, infective endocarditis, or rheumatic fever.

Pulmonary stenosis. Most commonly a congenital defect, pulmonary stenosis may also result from rheumatic fever, infective endocarditis, and trauma (rare).

The patient may be asymptomatic, or he may complain of dyspnea, fatigue, syncope, or chest pain. If the condition progresses, he may develop right heart failure. Auscultate for a harsh murmur in the pulmonic area. You may also hear a systolic thrill.

A pulmonary stenosis patient may require little treatment. If right ventricular failure develops, however, he may need a valvotomy or, in rare cases, pulmonic valve replacement.

Pulmonary insufficiency. This condition may be functional or organic. Functional causes include pulmonary artery hypertension or pulmonary artery dilation. Organic causes include infective endocarditis, trauma, and rheumatic fever.

Most patients with pulmonary insufficiency don't have symptoms unless right heart failure develops. Palpate for pulsation at the second left intercostal space. Also auscultate Erb's point for a diastolic murmur that intensifies on inspiration.

Interventions depend on the course of the underlying primary disease. The doctor may perform surgery if heart failure develops.

Valvular Heart Disease

Self Test

1. Which of the following ranks as your first care priority for the patient with suspected coronary artery disease (CAD)?
a. identifying risk factors   **b.** relieving anxiety   **c.** educating your patient about the disease process   **d.** enhancing myocardial oxygenation and perfusion

2. The stepped approach to stable angina treatment includes all of the following drugs, except:
a. vasodilators   **b.** nitrates   **c.** calcium channel blockers
d. beta blockers

3. Which serum enzyme test gives the most accurate indication of myocardial infarction (MI)?
a. CPK-MB   **b.** CPK-MM   **c.** LDH_1 **d.** LDH_2

4. Initial nursing goals for the patient with acute MI may include all of the following, except:
a. relieving pain   **b.** minimizing myocardial damage   **c.** improving tissue oxygenation   **d.** maximizing myocardial oxygen consumption

5. Which of these disorders most commonly complicates MI?
a. congestive heart failure   **b.** dysrhythmias   **c.** thromboembolism
d. ICU psychosis

6. Of the findings listed below, which one doesn't indicate left heart failure?
a. crackles   **b.** ventricular gallop (S_3)   **c.** elevated pulmonary capillary wedge pressure (PCWP)   **d.** dependent pitting peripheral edema

7. Heart failure may result from any of the following conditions, except:
a. increased metabolic demands   **b.** increased catecholamine release
c. abnormal muscle function   **d.** increased heart work load

8. When listening for heart sounds in a patient with pericarditis, you'll typically hear a:
a. systolic   murmur   **b.** diastolic   murmur   **c.** ejection   click
d. friction rub

9. Which of the following disorders commonly complicates myocarditis?
a. congestive heart failure   **b.** MI   **c.** pericarditis
d. cardiac tamponade

10. When assessing a patient with mitral valve prolapse, expect to hear a:
a. high-frequency click   **b.** low-frequency click   **c.** decrescendo murmur   **d.** crescendo-decrescendo murmur

11. A patient with acute aortic insufficiency may also show signs and symptoms of:
a. right-heart failure   **b.** pulmonary edema   **c.** tricuspid insufficiency
d. mitral insufficiency

Answers (page number shows where answer appears in text)

1. **d** (page 35)   2. **a** (page 48)   3. **a** (page 55)   4. **d** (page 58)
5. **b** (page 60)   6. **d** (page 68)   7. **b** (pages 64-65)   8. **d** (page 82)
9. **a** (page 92)   10. **a** (page 98)   11. **b** (page 100)

Dysrhythmias: Interruption of the Heart's Normal Rhythm

Mary Cooney, who wrote part of this chapter, is a staff nurse in the intensive cardiac care unit at Grandview Hospital, Sellersville, Pa. She received her ADN from Middlesex County College in Edison, N.J.

Margaret T. Perrone also contributed to this chapter. A staff nurse at the University of Michigan Hospitals in Ann Arbor, she earned her BSN from the University.

To care for a patient with a dysrhythmia, you need a thorough understanding of cardiac electrophysiology and its relationship to normal—and abnormal—cardiac function. Let's start by reviewing normal electrophysiology.

Myocardial cells have these four characteristics:
• *excitability*, the ability to respond to a stimulus
• *automaticity*, the ability to spontaneously initiate or propagate an action potential (usually a characteristic of pacemaker cells)
• *conductivity*, the ability to conduct the impulse to the next cell
• *contractility*, the ability to contract after depolarization.

A cell's ability to initiate or propagate an action potential varies during the repolarization/depolarization process. When the cell

Continued on page 104

Circus reentry

In this phenomenon (diagrammed below), an impulse delay takes place within a slow conduction pathway. Thus, the impulse remains active when the surrounding myocardium repolarizes. The impulse reenters the tissues and produces another impulse. Reentry may occur in any part of the myocardium or conduction system.

A reentry circuit can arise only when the following exist:
• a triggering impulse, either normal sinus or ectopic
• a slow conduction area that's long enough for the impulse traveling through to remain active after the remaining myocardial tissue becomes nonrefractory
• one-way conduction, preventing the impulse from cancelling itself out within the slow conduction area.

Another reentry type, *focal reentry*, results when repolarizing fibers reexcite fully repolarized fibers. This may occur when neighboring fibers simultaneously (or nearly simultaneously) become activated, but repolarize at different rates. This initiates the second beat.

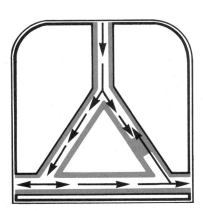

The conduction system: A quick review

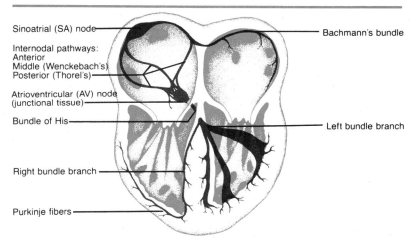

The heart's conduction system (shown above)—unique in its ability to spontaneously initiate and transmit electrical impulses—consists of the SA node, internodal tracts and Bachmann's bundle, AV node, bundle of His, right and left bundle branches, and the Purkinje fibers.

SA node and atrial conduction. Located in the right atrium where the superior vena cava joins the atrial tissue mass, the SA node serves as the heart's main pacemaker. Under resting conditions, the SA node initiates 60 to 100 beats/minute.

Internodal tracts and Bachmann's bundle. From the SA node, the impulse travels along three internodal tracts—the anterior, middle (Wenckebach), and posterior (Thorel's) tracts in the right atrium—and to the left atrium along Bachmann's bundle.

AV node. This node, situated in the right atrium between the coronary sinus and the tricuspid valve's septal cusp, doesn't possess pacemaker cells. However, the junctional tissue around it does. The AV node causes a brief (0.04 second) delay in electrical impulse conduction giving the atria time to contract. Rapid conduction then resumes through the bundle of His and down the left and right bundle branches.

The bundle of His. This pacemaker site, with an automatic firing rate between 40 and 60 beats/minute, divides into the right and left bundle branches. These branches extend down either side of the interventricular septum.

Purkinje's fibers. This diffuse muscle fiber network beneath the endocardium conducts impulses faster than any other cardiac region. Its automatic firing rate ranges from 15 to 40 beats/minute.

Conduction speed in the left bundle exceeds that in the right, giving the left ventricle's larger muscle mass the added time required to contract simultaneously with the right ventricle.

Dysrhythmias

Electrical before mechanical

Before the heart can mechanically contract and pump blood, cardiac muscle cell depolarization must take place. The exchange of sodium and potassium ions in myocardial cells creates electrical activity, which appears on the EKG as waveforms. Once depolarized and influenced by calcium ions, the cells mechanically contract (which you feel when taking a patient's pulse).

The *myocardial action potential curve* reflects this electrical activity. Here's what happens in each phase.

Phase 0: rapid depolarization. Sodium rapidly enters the cell while potassium leaves.

Phase 1: early rapid repolarization. With depolarization complete, this phase starts when potassium begins to reenter the cell and sodium begins to leave.

Phase 2: plateau. Penetrating the cell through the slow channels, calcium causes cellular contraction with sufficient time for a full contraction before another begins.

Phase 3: final rapid repolarization. The cell rapidly completes repolarization with sodium, and then calcium, pumped out of the cell and potassium pumped back in.

Phase 4: return to resting state. During this phase, the cell returns to its resting state. Sodium and calcium remain outside the cell; potassium, inside.

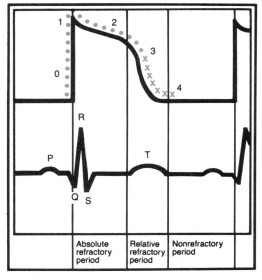

The graph (left) shows how the refractory period of the action potential curve corresponds to the EKG tracing.

Continued

reaches threshold, it can't respond to any stimulus, no matter how strong; this interval's called the *absolute refractory period*. As repolarization continues, however, the cell's responsiveness increases. During this time, called the *relative refractory* or *vulnerable period*, the cell can respond to a stimulus. (For more on action potential phases, see *Electrical before mechanical*, at left.)

Although myocardial cells generate impulses independently, they're influenced by both the sympathetic and parasympathetic divisions of the autonomic nervous system. Sympathetic fibers innervate all heart regions; parasympathetic fibers innervate the atria, sinoatrial (SA) node, atrioventricular (AV) node, and bifurcating bundle.

When stimulated, sympathetic fibers enhance excitability (bathomotropic effect), pacemaker firing rate (chronotropic effect), conduction speed (dromotropic effect) and contractility (inotropic effect). In contrast, parasympathetic stimulation depresses these effects.

Dysrhythmia causes. Dysrhythmias result from either an impulse formation disturbance or a conduction disturbance. Mechanisms that cause impulse formation disturbances include:
• altered automaticity. Enhanced automaticity may cause extrasystoles, premature beats, or tachycardias; depressed automaticity may lead to bradycardias or escape beats.
• afterdepolarization and triggered activity, resulting in repetitive ectopic firing from stimulation by a prior impulse.

Conduction disturbances result from:
• a conduction delay or block
• reentry (see *Circus reentry*, page 103).

Assessment

The patient history and physical assessment have limited value in identifying a specific dysrhythmia; only an electrocardiogram (EKG) can record the electrical activity that distinguishes one dysrhythmia from another. Nevertheless, assessment findings can provide information about your patient's condition as well as clues about the dysrhythmia type. Your findings may also help you identify related complications. In a patient with sinus tachycardia, for instance, you

Dysrhythmias

may note signs and symptoms of decreased cardiac output. For these reasons, never underestimate the value of a complete history and physical assessment. (For more information on assessment, review Chapter 1.)

Interpreting an EKG. Because the EKG provides the best information about dysrhythmias, you need to know how to interpret an EKG strip correctly. Read what follows for one of several methods you can use. *Remember:* The EKG provides information about just one aspect of your patient's condition. To intervene appropriately, consider *all* his needs.

To interpret an EKG strip, first estimate *heart rate* by counting the number of QRS complexes in a 6-second strip and multiplying by 10. To determine ventricular rate, count the number of R waves; determine atrial rate by counting the number of P waves. Use this method for a strip with irregular RR and PP intervals.

If an R wave falls on one of the heavier dark lines, estimate ventricular rate by counting the numbers 300, 150, 100, 75, 60, and 50 for each heavy line that follows, until you see the next heavy

Continued on page 106

Reviewing EKG basics

The electrocardiogram (EKG) reflects the electrical acitvity of cardiac cells. With the aid of a hot stylus, the EKG machine records this activity onto heat-sensitive paper running at a speed of 25 mm/second.

An EKG strip consists of horizontal squares representing seconds and vertical squares representing voltage. Each small square (shown by lighter lines) represents 0.04 second or 0.1 mV (1mm). Each large square (shown by heavy lines) represents 0.20 second or 0.5 mV (5mm). (*Note:* 0.04 second equals 40 milliseconds.)

An EKG waveform (see illustration at right) has three basic elements: P wave, QRS complex, and T wave. These elements can be further divided into a PR interval, U wave, ST segment, J point and QT interval. Let's take a closer look at each.

• The **P wave** represents atrial depolarization.

• The **PR interval** represents the time it takes an impulse to travel from the atria through the AV node, bundle of His, and bundle branches to the Purkinje fibers. Measure the PR interval from the beginning of the P wave to the beginning of the QRS complex. Normal PR interval duration ranges from 0.12 to 0.20 second.

• The **QRS complex** represents ventricular depolarization. Mea-

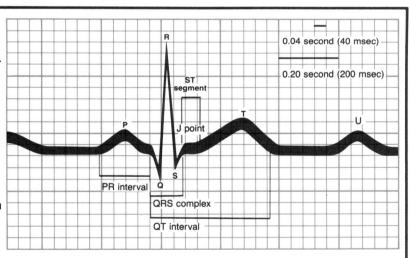

sured from the beginning to the end of the QRS complex, this normally lasts for 0.06 to 0.10 second. (Because the ventricles depolarize quickly, reducing the contact time between the stylus and EKG paper, the QRS complex usually appears thinner than other EKG elements.)

The **Q wave** appears as the first negative deflection in the QRS complex; the **R wave**, as the first positive deflection. The **S wave** appears as the second negative deflection, or the first negative deflection after the R wave. (Keep in mind, however, that you may not see all three QRS complex waves.)

Atrial repolarization usually takes place during this time, but the QRS complex obscures it on the EKG.

• The **J point** marks the end of the QRS complex and the beginning of the ST segment.

• The **ST segment** represents part of ventricular repolarization. This line usually appears slightly positive.

• The **T wave** represents ventricular repolarization. This usually follows the same deflection pattern as the QRS complex.

• The **U wave** follows the T wave. A prominent U wave may indicate an electrolyte abnormality.

• The **QT interval** represents ventricular refractory time. It extends from the beginning of the QRS complex to the end of the T wave. It normally lasts 0.36 to 0.44 second, but varies with the patient's heart rate, age, and sex.

Dysrhythmias

Continued

line with an R wave. The last number you count shows an estimated ventricular rate. *Note:* You can use this method to estimate atrial rate, if a P wave falls on a heavy line.

If R waves occur at regular intervals, you can more accurately estimate ventricular rate by counting the number of large boxes in an RR interval, then dividing that number into 300 (the number of 0.20-second boxes in a 1-minute strip).

Next, answer these questions:
• Is the rhythm regular or irregular?
• Do you see P waves?
• Do P waves have a normal shape—upright and rounded? Abnormally shaped P waves suggest that the impulse originated in atrial or junctional tissue rather than in the sinus node.
• Do you see a one-to-one relationship between P waves and QRS complexes? This indicates sinus impulse conduction to the ventricles.
• Does the PR interval fall within normal limits (0.12 to 0.20 second)? This indicates normal impulse conduction.
• Does the time interval between QRS complexes fall within normal limits (0.06 to 0.10 second)?
• Do you see T waves? If so, do they point in the same direction as the QRS complex? Do they have a normal shape?
• Does the QT interval fall within normal limits (0.36 to 0.44 second)?
• Do you see ectopic or aberrantly conducted beats?

If you were using the preceding method to evaluate an EKG strip showing a normal sinus rhythm, here's what you'd find: atrial and ventricular rates between 60 and 100 beats/minute; regular rhythm; a normally shaped P wave preceding each QRS complex; and PR intervals and QRS complexes falling within normal limits. You wouldn't see any ectopic or aberrantly conducted impulses.

Normal sinus rhythm

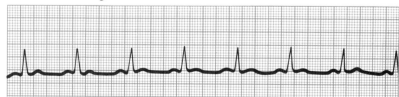

Other EKG types. By inserting an electrode into the esophagus (which lies next to the posterior atria), the doctor can obtain an esophageal EKG strip that's diagnostic of certain dysrhythmias, particularly supraventricular dysrhythmias. He may also use the electrode for atrial and even ventricular pacing.

To assess atrial activity and its relationship to ventricular activity, he may use an atrial EKG. For this diagnostic test, he inserts temporary atrial epicardial wires during cardiac surgery. Or, he may insert temporary atrial electrodes transvenously.

Identifying electrolyte imbalances. Your patient's EKG strip can alert you to abnormal serum potassium and calcium levels—common dysrhythmia causes. In the case of hyperkalemia, EKG changes provide clues to the degree of imbalance. Watch for the following.

Dysrhythmias

Cardiac monitor lead placements

These illustrations show the EKG electrode placements for three commonly used leads.

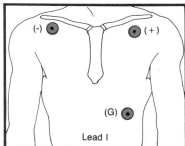

Lead I

Lead I
Positive (+): left shoulder, below clavicular hollow
Negative (−): right shoulder, below clavicular hollow
Ground (G): left side of chest, lowest palpable rib, midclavicular line

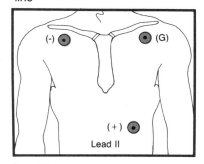

Lead II

Lead II
Positive (+): left side of chest, lowest palpable rib, midclavicular line
Negative (−): right shoulder, below clavicular hollow
Ground (G): left shoulder, below clavicular hollow

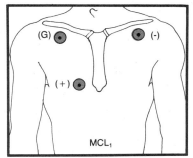

MCL₁

MCL₁
Positive (+): fourth ICS, right sternal border (V_1 position)
Negative (−): left shoulder, below clavicular hollow
Ground (G): right shoulder, below clavicular hollow

Important: Don't place leads directly over bony areas such as the ribs.

- *Serum potassium level between 5.5 and 6.5 mEq/l:* Tented T waves (tall, peaked T waves with a narrow base).
- *Serum potassium level between 6.5 and 8.0 mEq/l:* Decreased R wave amplitude; increased S wave depth; prolonged QRS complexes; lengthened PR intervals; flattened P waves; tented T waves; ventricular dysrhythmias.
- *Serum potassium level above 8.0 mEq/l:* Loss of atrial activity (sinus impulses may continue to reach the ventricles via internodal tracts); marked QRS widening; T wave inversion or disappearance; merging of QRS complexes and inverted T waves (similar to "dying heart" configuration); complete heart block; ventricular tachycardia or fibrillation; asystole.
- *Serum potassium level below 3.5 mEq/l:* Flattened or notched T waves; pronounced U waves; prolonged QT interval; premature ventricular contractions; ST segment depression.
- *Serum calcium level above 16 mg/dl:* Shortened QT interval; sagging, shortened ST interval; inverted T waves; ventricular dysrhythmias.
- *Serum calcium level below 6.1 mg/dl:* Prolonged QT interval and ST segment duration; flattened or inverted T waves.

Electrophysiology (EP) studies. With the aid of an EP study, an intracardiac EKG procedure, the doctor can assess drug therapy, locate ectopic foci and bypass tracts (as in preexcitation syndromes), and determine the need for a pacemaker or surgery. Because intracardiac EP catheters lie closer to the cardiac conduction system than do an EKG's external electrodes, EP studies give more detailed information about the heart's electrical activity.

To assess drug therapy, the doctor follows this procedure: First, he places intracardiac catheters and pacing wires transvenously (to study the right heart) or transarterially (to study the left heart). Next, he stimulates extrasystolic beats and induces ventricular tachycardia. Then, he gives various I.V. antiarrhythmic drugs and evaluates their ability to control the dysrhythmia. A drug that controls an induced dysrhythmia may prevent or control a similar spontaneous dysrhythmia.

To locate ectopic foci, the doctor uses EP in conjunction with a technique called *mapping*. First, he divides the heart into imaginary sections and assigns each section a number. Then, he systematically stimulates each section until he induces a dysrhythmia. Once he's pinpointed the dysrhythmia's origin, he can proceed with ablation or another surgical procedure, if indicated.

If the patient has supraventricular tachycardia accompanied by syncope uncontrolled by drug therapy, the doctor may order EP testing to identify the underlying mechanism. The procedure can also help the doctor differentiate wide-complex tachycardias (such as ventricular and supraventricular tachycardia), enabling him to initiate appropriate therapy.

If your patient's scheduled for an EP procedure, document the presence and quality of peripheral pulses, to provide a baseline for postprocedure assessment. As ordered, discontinue antiarrhythmic drugs.

Tell the patient what to expect before, during, and after the pro-

Continued on page 108

Dysrhythmias

Continued

cedure. For example, tell him the procedure usually takes from 2 to 4 hours. Also explain that he may briefly lose consciousness if the doctor induces tachycardia; assure him that the doctor will quickly treat this expected effect. Tell him that he must keep the affected limb straight and still for about 8 hours afterwards.

After the procedure, regularly check vital signs and peripheral pulses (particularly those distal to the insertion site). Also check the insertion site for bleeding, hematoma, and inflammation.

His bundle studies. To locate the source of a heart block (particularly when appropriate therapy hinges on this information), the doctor may perform a His bundle study. This electrophysiologic study can also help him locate a reentrant pathway in a patient with pre-excitation syndrome. Follow the same teaching and nursing care guidelines provided for EP studies.

Planning

Care priorities include maintaining adequate cardiac output and preventing complications. See the sample care plan below for a generalized listing of expected outcomes, nursing interventions, and discharge planning for a patient with a dysrhythmia. However, remember to individualize each care plan according to the needs of the patient and his family. As always, focus on caring for the patient—not the dysrhythmia. (For the clinical implications of each dysrhythmia type, see the second part of this chapter.)

Nursing diagnoses. Possible nursing diagnoses for a patient with a dysrhythmia include:
• cardiac output, alteration in (decreased), potential for; related to cardiac dysrhythmia
• fluid volume, alteration in (excess), potential for; related to dysrhythmia
• tissue perfusion, alteration in, potential for; related to dysrhythmia

---

Sample nursing care plan—dysrhythmia

Nursing diagnosis	**Expected outcomes**
Cardiac output, alteration in (decreased), potential for; related to cardiac dysrhythmia	The patient will: • maintain adequate cardiac output • maintain adequate tissue and myocardial perfusion • show knowledge of signs and symptoms of decreased cardiac output.
Nursing interventions • Determine dysrhythmia type and its potential for decreasing cardiac output. • Maintain continuous dysrhythmia monitoring in EKG lead that best reveals the patient's dysrhythmia. • Observe for changes in dysrhythmia. • Document the dysrhythmia type. • Monitor vital signs, level of consciousness, urinary output, and any chest pain; these may indicate decreased cardiac output. • Teach patient about signs and symptoms of decreased cardiac output. Make sure he knows when to notify you or the doctor.	**Discharge planning** • Teach patient about his dysrhythmia. • Reinforce need to advise doctor of signs or symptoms of decreased cardiac output. • Teach patient when to seek medical care. • Arrange for follow-up doctor's visit.

Dysrhythmias

- activity intolerance; related to dysrhythmia
- breathing patterns, ineffective (shortness of breath); related to dysrhythmia
- knowledge deficit; related to dysrhythmia and underlying disease process
- noncompliance, potential for; related to inadequate health teaching
- anxiety; related to dysrhythmia and underlying disease process.

Interventions

Dysrhythmia treatments may vary significantly, depending on the patient's condition. One patient might not need any treatment; another might require drug therapy or surgery.

Drug therapy. If the patient needs drug therapy, the choice of drug depends on what type of dysrhythmia he has, where it arises in the heart, and what signs and symptoms he has. Let's take a closer look.

Most antiarrhythmic drugs are classified according to their effects—direct or indirect—on the action potential's duration.
- *Class I antiarrhythmics*, which affect fast (sodium) channels, contain two subgroups. Drugs in the first subgroup—quinidine, procainamide, and disopyramide—slow the sodium channel, which normally allows cardiac cells to depolarize quickly. These antiarrhythmics allow fewer sodium ions to pass through the cardiac membrane at a time, thus prolonging the time a cell needs to completely depolarize. They also increase the absolute refractory period (preventing cells from responding immediately to another stimulus) and depress Purkinje fiber automaticity. On EKG, these effects appear as a slightly widened QRS complex and a prolonged QT interval. Quinidine and procainamide may also produce U waves and cause T waves to flatten or invert.

Lidocaine, phenytoin, and tocainide represent the second subgroup of Class I antiarrhythmics. These drugs, which more strongly affect diseased myocardial tissue than healthy tissue, control ventricular dysrhythmias and decrease ventricular conduction cell automaticity. Although no one fully understands why these drugs work, they may shorten the refractory period in Purkinje and ventricular muscle cells. On EKG, they may slightly shorten the QT interval.
- *Class II antiarrhythmics* (beta-adrenergic blockers) include propranolol (Inderal), nadalol, timolol, atenolol, and metoprolol. These drugs reduce the effects of circulating catecholamines. Beta-one sites primarily affect the heart; beta-two sites, bronchial and vascular smooth muscle tissue. They also slow SA nodal impulses. Drug effects include decreased heart rate and vasodilation (which lowers blood pressure) thereby reducing the heart's oxygen requirements. Some evidence suggests that beta blockers reduce the risk of sudden death from ventriculr fibrillation in post-MI patients.

Use caution when giving a beta blocker to a patient with left ventricular dysfunction; a beta blocker may exacerbate heart failure. And don't give a beta blocker to a patient with asthma; its effects on beta-two receptor sites may lead to bronchoconstriction and spasm.
- *Class III antiarrhythmics* include bretylium and amiodarone (as well as other drugs under investigation). These agents control su-

Handwritten margin notes:

CLASS Ia: Quinidine
   Procainamide
   Disopyramide
   ↓(fast) Na⁺ Channels ∴ ↑depol time
   ↑absolute Refractory Time
   depress Purkinjie Fib Automaticity.
EKG Δ's: slight widen of QRS
   prolonged QT
   ∈ Quin ε Proc: ⇒ U waves
      Flatten or Invert T.

CLASS Ib: LIDOCAINE
   PHENYTOIN
   TOCAINIDE
   more affect on diseased tissue
CONTROL VENT DYSRYTHMS
   by ↓ VENT CONDUCTION
   CELL AUTOMATICITY
   ⇒ by shortening Refract. In Purk.
      ε vent muscle cells
ECK Δ's: ⇒ slight shorten QT

CLASS II (B-Adrenergic blockers)
   PROPRANOLOL (INDERAL)

Continued on page 110

Dysrhythmias

Continued

praventricular and ventricular dysrhythmias by increasing the refractory period and action potential duration without affecting conduction time or depressing cardiac contractility. They may also control ventricular dysrhythmias that don't respond to other drugs. On EKG, expect these drugs to cause QRS widening, bradycardia, and prolonged QT intervals.

• *Class IV antiarrhythmics* (calcium channel blockers) include verapamil, diltiazem, and nifedipine. They affect slow (calcium) channels that predominate in arterial smooth muscle and nodal tissue. Except for nifedipine, these drugs help control supraventricular tachycardias (especially those involving the AV node) because they inhibit AV node conduction.

Nifedipine has a stronger effect on arterial smooth muscle than on nodal tissue. Because it dilates peripheral arteries, it's used primarily as an antihypertensive drug. Like other class IV drugs, it also helps relieve angina pain secondary to coronary spasm.

Nursing considerations. If your patient's undergoing antiarrhythmic drug therapy, document his apical heart rate and blood pressure before giving each drug dose. Evaluate a rhythm strip at least once every 4 hours; if you see any changes (or if the patient becomes symptomatic), notify the doctor and obtain a 12-lead EKG, as ordered. Also monitor laboratory values (including serum electrolyte and drug levels) for signs of complications. Document all nursing actions you take.

In addition, teach the patient and his family about his drug regimen and stress the importance of compliance. Work out a convenient schedule that ensures drug effectiveness. Also discuss possible adverse drug effects with the patient, and advise him to call the doctor or nurse if he experiences effects or symptoms of dysrhythmia (lightheadedness, dizziness, palpitations, or weakness).

Electrosurgery. If a ventricular dysrhythmia doesn't respond to drug therapy or pacing techniques (which we'll discuss shortly), the doctor may perform surgery to excise the site of ectopic foci or a reentrant pathway. Before surgery, he localizes the site with ventricular mapping (see page 107). With the help of preoperative cardiac catheterization, he assesses the patient's hemodynamic status, ventricular function, and coronary artery blood flow.

To excise the site, the doctor can choose one of several techniques.
• *Endocardial excision* requires open heart surgery and cardiopulmonary bypass. The doctor penetrates the ventricle (usually through an aneurysm or scar tissue from a past infarction) and removes the ectopic foci site, along with tissue extending 2 cm on each side of it, by peeling the endocardium.
• *Cryosurgery* ablates the involved tissue by freezing, which destroys only a small portion of normal tissue. The method doesn't require open-heart surgery. Because the procedure causes a small infarction, care for the postcryosurgical patient as you would an MI patient.
• *Thermal ablation* destroys the site by burning. Most often used to correct refractory ventricular tachydysrhythmias and accessory pathways secondary to preexcitation syndrome, this procedure can be performed in the EP laboratory.

Dysrhythmias

Pacemaker glossary

capture: a pacemaker's ability to cause atrial and/or ventricular depolarization.

hysteresis: a programmable feature; the pacemaker escape interval (the period between an intrinsic beat and the next paced beat).

MA (milliamperes): the amount of current needed to elicit myocardial depolarization (0.1 to 20 MA).

pacing artifact (spike): the thin EKG line that indicates pacemaker firing.

sense: a pacemaker's ability to detect atrial and/or ventricular depolarization.

sensitivity (millivolts): the voltage required to deliver the current (0.5 to 20 mV).

threshold: the amount of electrical current or voltage needed to elicit depolarization and, thus, cause contraction.

Before, during, and after the procedure, your nursing responsibilities include patient teaching and providing emotional support.

Pacemakers. The doctor may recommend an artificial pacemaker to stimulate myocardial cell depolarization and effective contraction. A *demand* pacemaker senses intrinsic cardiac rhythm and stimulates myocardial depolarization and contraction as necessary. A *fixed-rate* pacemaker fires at a predetermined rate, regardless of intrinsic cardiac activity.

All pacemakers have two basic components: a pulse generator, containing a power source and electronic circuitry; and one or two pacing leads, each with an electrode on its tip. Pacemakers can be either temporary or permanent, depending on whether the pulse generator's external or implanted. Here's how the two types compare.

A temporary pacemaker may be used for a patient experiencing syncope of unknown cause or signs and symptoms related to bradycardia, tachycardia, MI, or heart block. If the patient's asymptomatic, the doctor considers the patient's resting EKG, prognosis, and general condition before deciding whether to use a temporary pacemaker.

The doctor can insert temporary pacemaker leads into the right ventricle in several ways: transvenously, transthoracically (through closed-chest puncture), or via a five-lumen pulmonary artery catheter. Or he can insert insulated wires (epicardial leads) during open-heart surgery.

Most temporary pacemakers have bipolar leads. Both electrodes (located several millimeters apart) rest in the heart; both sense spontaneous cardiac activity; one stimulates the heart.

The pacemaker's pulse generator, which remains outside the body, has dial or touch controls. Most generators run on ordinary alkaline batteries. *Note:* In an emergency, the doctor may use a noninvasive

Continued on page 113

Recognizing pacemaker spikes

The pacemaker sends an electrical impulse to the heart, which appears on the EKG strip as a vertical line, commonly called the pacemaker spike. A spike followed by a QRS complex or P wave shows that *capture* has occurred.

If the pacemaker electrode rests in the ventricle, you'll see a spike in front of every QRS complex stimulated by the pacemaker. These complexes appear wide and bizarre—similar to those caused by premature ventricular contractions, except that they won't be early. If the electrode's in the atrium, a spike before a P wave indicates capture's occurred; the P wave may be inverted or may differ in shape from a spontaneous P wave. If electrodes pace both the atria and ventricles, you'll see spikes before both QRS complexes and P waves.

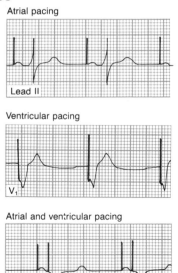

Atrial pacing

Lead II

Ventricular pacing

V₁

Atrial and ventricular pacing

V₁

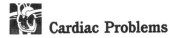

Dysrhythmias

Reviewing pacemaker codes

A pacemaker coding system devised by the Intersociety Commission for Heart Disease (ICHD) clearly identifies pacemaker capabilities. The code's five letters have the following significance.

• The first letter signifies the heart chamber being paced: A (atrium), V (ventricle), or D (dual, or both chambers).

• The second letter identifies the heart chamber the pacemaker senses: A, V, D, or O (none or not applicable).

• The third letter indicates how the pacemaker generator responds to the sensed event: T (triggered), I (inhibited), D (both triggered and inhibited), or O (not applicable).

• The fourth letter shows the number of available reprogrammable functions.

• The fifth letter indicates how the pacemaker reacts to tachycardia.

Keep in mind, though, that most pacemakers codes only refer to the first three letters. Consider this when reviewing the chart below, which describes pacemaker indications, advantages, and disadvantages.

Mode
AAI, AAT
Indications
SSS with intact AV conduction
Advantages
• Simplest system that provides sequential AV depolarization
• Requires single lead

• Easily understood function
Disadvantages
• Won't pace ventricle if AV block develops
• Inhibits atrial impulses by sensing QRS complexes

Mode
VVI, VVT
Indications
• Atrial flutter or fibrillation, or multifocal atrial tachycardia with slow ventricular response
• Infrequent bradycardia
• Insufficient hemodynamic response to AV sequential pacing
• Recurrent pacemaker-mediated tachycardia (PMT)
Advantages
• Requires single lead
• Relatively simple to operate
Disadvantages
• Doesn't change rate in response to increased metabolic demands
• Doesn't preserve AV synchrony
• May cause retrograde AV conduction and echo beats
• May cause pacemaker syndrome

Mode
VAT
Indications
• Obsolete, but available as programmable function mode
Advantages
• None
Disadvantages
• May cause competitive ventricular rhythms from lack of ventricular sensing

Mode
VDD
Indications
• Impaired AV conduction with normal sinus node function
Advantages
• Maintains AV synchrony and rate responsiveness to increased metabolic demands when atrial rate

stays within tracking limits
Disadvantages
• Requires two leads
• Doesn't pace atrium
• May cause PMT
• Lacks AV synchrony and rate responsiveness during atrial bradycardia

Mode
DVI
Indications
• Atrial bradycardia
• PMT in VDD and DDD modes
Advantages
• Maintains AV synchrony during atrial bradycardia
• Permits AV rate control to decrease myocardial oxygen demands during angina
• Lack of atrial sensing may prevent PMT
Disadvantages
• Requires two leads
• Doesn't maintain AV synchrony unless pacemaker's programmed automatic rate exceeds spontaneous atrial rate
• Doesn't change rate in response to increased metabolic needs
• May cause competitive atrial rhythms from lack of atrial sensing

Mode
DDD
Indications
• Atrial bradydysrhythmia
• Normal sinus node function with abnormal AV conduction
Advantages
• Maintains AV synchrony
• Most closely mimics normal cardiac physiology
Disadvantages
• Requires two leads
• Most complex design
• May cause PMT
• Paced rate doesn't increase to meet metabolic demands if sinus node dysfunction occurs, unless programmed to do so

Guide to pacemaker codes

Letter position				
1 Chamber paced	2 Chamber sensed	3 Mode of response	4 Programmable functions	5 Tachydysrhythmia function
Letters used				
V:Ventricle	V:Ventricle	T:Triggered	P: Programmable (rate and/or output only)	B:Bursts
A:Atrium	A:Atrium	I:Inhibited	M: Multi-programmable	N: Normal rate competition
D:Double	D:Double	D:Double O:None	C: Communicating	S:Scanning
	O:None	R:Reverse	O:None	E:External

Dysrhythmias

Continued

transcutaneous temporary pacemaker, which stimulates the heart through electrodes placed on the patient's chest and back.

A permanent pacemaker may have either a bipolar or unipolar lead system. In a unipolar system, one electrode rests in the heart; the pulse generator contains a second (indifferent) electrode. (Some permanent pacemakers can be programmed to either a unipolar or bipolar system.) Most permanent pacemakers run on lithium batteries.

As a rule, the doctor gives the patient a local anesthetic and inserts the pacemaker lead transvenously in the catheterization laboratory, special procedures department, or operating room. After inserting the lead into the chamber, he anchors it in the endocardial trabeculae by means of a flange-tine or fin-tipped device, spring-released barb, screw, or clamp at the lead's tip. Then he implants the pulse generator in a subcutaneous pocket, usually under the clavicle, or in some cases, under the abdominal wall.

Programmed when inserted, most permanent pacemakers can be easily reprogrammed if the patient's needs change after insertion. For example, heart rate or refractory period, can be altered by noninvasive transmission of information from an external programmer to the implanted generator.

Indications for permanent pacing include:
• asymptomatic sinus pauses longer than 2.5 seconds or sinus bradycardia with rates less than 40 beats/minute (unless the patient's a conditioned athlete)
• symptomatic second-degree AV heart block
• anterior MI with first-degree AV block and right bundle branch block with left atrial hypertrophy
• asymptomatic complete AV block with a rate less than 40 beats/minute
• hereditary, idiopathic, or drug-related QT interval prolongation
• vasovagal bradycardia with syncope.

Patient care. When caring for a pacemaker patient, your responsibilities include assessing pacemaker function, maintaining system integrity, ensuring patient safety and comfort, preventing complications, and teaching the patient about his condition and treatment. (See pages 114 and 115 for details on troubleshooting pacemakers.)

Evaluation

Base your evaluation on the type of dysrhythmia the patient has and the expected outcomes listed on his nursing care plan. Using the sample care plan on page 108 as a guide, for example, you might ask yourself the following questions:
• Can the patient maintain adequate cardiac output for tissue and myocardial perfusion?
• Does he know the signs and symptoms of decreased cardiac output?
• Does he know when to seek medical attention for these signs and symptoms?

The answers to these questions will help you evaluate your patient's status and the effectiveness of his care. Keep in mind that these questions stem from the sample care plan. Your questions may differ.

Dysrhythmias

Troubleshooting pacemakers

When your patient's pacemaker malfunctions, taking a systematic approach will help you identify and correct the problem. Begin by answering the following questions:
- Is the pacemaker temporary or permanent?
- What's the pacemaker's mode (for example, DVI or DDD)?
- What's the programmed rate?
- Does it pace or capture appropriately?
- Does it sense appropriately?
- Does the patient have signs and symptoms?

(*Note:* Placing a magnet over the permanent pacemaker may help pinpoint the problem.)

The chart that follows provides guidelines for identifying and dealing with some common pacemaker problems.

Failure to capture

Signs and symptoms
- Bradycardia
- Hypotension
- Fatigue
- EKG pacemaker spikes not followed by QRS complexes (if the pacemaker uses a ventricular electrode) or by P waves (if it uses an atrial electrode)

Possible causes
- Electrode tip out of position
- Pacemaker voltage too low
- Lead wire fracture
- Battery depletion
- Edema or scar tissue formation at electrode tip
- Myocardial perforation by lead wire

Interventions
- Reposition electrode tip
- Increase voltage (MA)
- Replace lead
- Replace battery
- Reposition or replace lead

- Surgery

Failure to pace

Signs and symptoms
- No apparent pacemaker activity on EKG
- Hypotension
- Bradycardia
- Magnet application yields no response

Possible causes
- Battery failure
- Circuitry failure
- Lead displacement or fracture
- Broken or loose lead-generator connection

Interventions
- Replace battery
- Replace generator
- Replace lead
- Repair connection (for a temporary pacemaker, tighten terminal)

Failure to sense (competition or undersensing)

Signs and symptoms
- Palpitations
- Skipped beats
- Ventricular tachycardia
- EKG pacemaker spikes that fall where they shouldn't; spikes may fall on T waves

Possible causes
- Battery depletion
- Electrode tip out of position

- Lead wire fracture
- Increased sensing threshold from edema or fibrosis at electrode tip

Interventions
- Replace battery
- Reposition electrode, or reposition patient by placing him on his left side
- Replace lead
- Adjust sensitivity setting
Important: Make sure undersensing's the true problem; some pacemakers (for example, the DDD type) may be programmed *not* to sense in a given time period.

Oversensing

Signs and symptoms
- Pacemaker paces at a rate slower than the set rate
- No paced beats (even though pacemaker's set rate exceeds patient's spontaneous rate)

Possible causes
- Myopotentials (with unipolar leads only). The pacemaker may sense (or be inhibited by) skeletal muscle contractions.
- Electromagnetic interference
- Sensing of T waves or atrial activity
- Pacemaker sensitivity set too high

Interventions
- Adjust sensitivity setting, insert bipolar lead

- Test with magnet, as ordered
- Adjust sensitivity setting

- Adjust sensitivity setting

Pacing at altered rate

Signs and symptoms
- Pacemaker spikes that don't occur at set rate (a "runaway" pacemaker may occur with pacing spikes at high rates, such as 150 to 180 beats/minute). Watch for signs and symptoms of decreased cardiac output and R-on-T phenomenon.

Possible causes
- Battery depletion
- Generator failure
- Phantom programming (pacemaker reprogrammed by source other than pacemaker programmer, such as electrocautery or Welder's arc)

Interventions
- Replace battery
- Replace generator
- Remove cause and reprogram pacemaker

Dysrhythmias

Premature ventricular contractions

Signs and symptoms
- Patient complains of skipped beats
- PVCs visible on EKG

Possible causes
- Electrode causing irritable ventricular focus. *Note:* PVCs occur normally in the first 24 hours after pacemaker insertion; they're not treated during this time unless they cause signs or symptoms.

Interventions
- Administer antiarrhythmic drugs, as ordered
- Reposition lead

Diaphragmatic or phrenic nerve stimulation

Signs and symptoms
- Hiccups
- EKG artifact

Possible causes
- Stimulation of phrenic nerve by electrode tip
- Myocardial perforation by lead wire
- Excessive pacemaker voltage (MAs)

Interventions
- Position patient on his side
- Surgery
- Decrease voltage (MAs)

Chest or abdominal muscle stimulation (muscle twitch)

Signs and symptoms
- Muscle twitching
- Pacemaker identification letters appear backward on chest X-ray

Possible causes
- High pacemaker output
- Lead fracture or insulation break
- Flipped pulse generator

Interventions
- Reduce pacemaker output
- Replace lead
- Reposition generator; instruct patient not to rub skin over pacemaker

Pacemaker syndrome
(loss of AV synchrony resulting in decreased cardiac output)

Signs and symptoms
- Weakness
- Decreased exercise tolerance
- Persistent unmanageable congestive heart failure

Possible causes
- Loss of atrioventricular (AV) synchrony in VVI or VVT pacing

Interventions
- Increase paced rate, if patient lacks intrinsic rhythm; decrease paced rate, if the intrinsic rhythm's adequate
- Suggest that the doctor replace pacemaker with a dual-chamber type that has atrial sensing (such as a DDD)

Pacemaker-mediated tachycardia (PMT)

Signs and symptoms
- Tachycardia with pacemaker spike preceding each QRS complex seen on EKG

Possible causes
- Retrograde conduction through AV node (from dual-chamber pacing such as DDD), which repolarizes atria and triggers rapid heart rate

Interventions
- Observe patient for ventricular tachycardia and fibrillation. The doctor or specially trained nurse will reprogram pacemaker to atrial nonsensing mode.
- In emergency, decrease heart rate by holding a magnet over pulse generator; this converts demand pacemaker into fixed pacemaker until it can be reprogrammed.

Specific dysrhythmias

Dysrhythmias usually result from disturbed impulse formation or conduction. Here's a closer look at the dysrhythmias you're most likely to encounter.

Sinus dysrhythmias
Sinus tachycardia

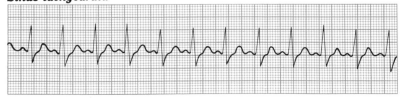

EKG characteristics. Normal rhythm; rate between 100 and 160 beats/minute.

Continued on page 116

Dysrhythmias

Reviewing dysrhythmia terms

aberrant: abnormal.

automatic beat: an impulse arising in an automatic focus, independent of dominant rhythm.

AV dissociation: the independent beating of atria and ventricles.

block: a pathologic delay or interruption in impulse conduction.

bradydysrhythmia: any rhythm disturbance causing a slow heart or chamber rate (less than 60 beats/minute).

coupling: the relationship of a premature beat to the beat preceding it.

coupling interval: the interval between a premature beat and the preceding beat.

ectopic beat: a beat that originates in a focus other than the normal sinus pacemaker.

electromechanical dissociation: electrical activity without evidence of myocardial contraction.

escape beat: an automatic beat that occurs after an interval longer than the dominant cycle.

extrasystole: an ectopic beat, occurring before the next dominant beat, that depends on and couples with the preceding beat.

fusion beat: simultaneous activation of one chamber by two foci.

group beating: a pattern of repetitive QRS complexes.

idiojunctional rhythm: a relatively slow, independent rhythm that arises in the AV junction and controls only the ventricles.

idioventricular rhythm: a relatively slow rhythm that originates from and controls the ventricles.

parasystole: an ectopic, independent rhythm that operates concurrently with the dominant rhythm, whose foci can't be discharged by dominant pacemaker impulses.

tachydysrhythmia: any rhythm disturbance resulting in a fast heart or chamber rate (over 100 beats/minute).

Specific dysrhythmias—*continued*

Clinical implications. This dysrhythmia, which shortens diastole, commonly arises from decreased vagal tone, increased sympathetic tone, digitalis toxicity, or increased oxygen demand (caused, for example, by fever, hypovolemia, anemia, exercise, or stress). In healthy people, caffeine, nicotine, or alcohol ingestion may trigger sinus tachycardia.

After an MI, sinus tachycardia may develop as a normal part of the inflammatory response. If prolonged, however, it's an ominous sign of congestive heart failure.

Interventions. These focus on correcting the underlying cause.

Sinus bradycardia

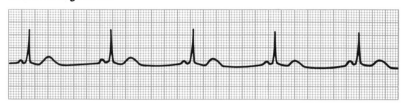

EKG characteristics. Normal rhythm; rate less than 60 beats/minute.

Clinical implications. In athletes, sinus bradycardia frequently develops because the well-conditioned heart can maintain stroke volume with less effort. Other possible causes include drug therapy (such as digitalis and beta blockers), severe pain, hyperkalemia, and vagal stimulation (occurring, for example, when the patient strains to pass stool). This dysrhythmia commonly arises after an inferior MI involving the right coronary artery, which supplies blood to the SA node.

Signs and symptoms include fatigue, light-headedness, syncope, and palpitations (because the SA node's increased relative refractory period permits ectopic firing). However, the patient may not experience these if he can compensate hemodynamically.

Interventions. The doctor won't usually treat this dysrhythmia unless it causes signs or symptoms. In that case, he'll order therapy aimed at correcting the underlying cause and maintain heart rate with drugs (such as atropine or isoproterenol) or a pacemaker.

Sinus arrhythmia

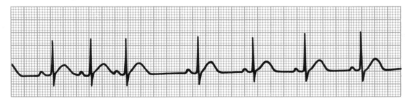

EKG characteristics. Normal rhythm, and varying PP intervals.

Clinical implications. Usually considered normal, this rhythm variation related to the respiratory cycle results from reflex vagal tone inhibition. The PP interval shortens during inspiration (increasing heart rate) and lengthens during expiration (decreasing rate). In rhythm variations not related to respiration, however, this dys-

Dysrhythmias

rhythmia probably arises from an underlying condition that increases vagal tone, such as digitalis toxicity, increased intracranial pressure, or inferior-wall MI. In the elderly, a marked variation in PP intervals may indicate sick sinus syndrome.

Interventions. The doctor will usually treat only patients who develop signs or symptoms. He may order a drug (such as atropine) to increase heart rate while treating the underlying cause.

Sinus block (SA block)

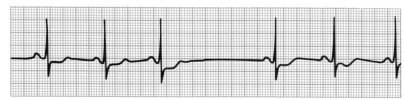

In all categories of SA block (first, second, and third degree), the pacemaker discharges at regular intervals, but the impulse is delayed or blocked from reaching the atria. Possible causes include any condition that increases vagal tone, hypersensitive carotid sinus, coronary artery disease (CAD), heart infections, and digitalis toxicity.

EKG characteristics. First-degree block: not diagnosable on EKG.

Second-degree Type I (Wenckebach) SA block: progressive PP interval shortening and a pause that's less than twice the initial PP interval. QRS complexes usually appear in a clearly repetitive pattern (group beating).

Second-degree Type II (Mobitz) SA block: a sudden dropped P wave—no P wave where you'd expect the next one to appear. The pause occurs in a cycle that's an interval of the usual PP cycle.

Third-degree SA block: long sinus pauses (absent P waves).

Clinical implications. First-degree block may result from delayed conduction either internodally or at the SA junction. Second-degree Type I block involves a progressive increase in conduction time through the SA node. Second-degree Type II block results when the SA node fails to initiate or conduct an impulse. Third-degree block results from failure of the SA node to initiate or discharge more than one impulse.

Interventions. An asymptomatic patient needs no treatment. If symptoms develop, however, the doctor treats bradycardia and the underlying cause.

Sinus arrest

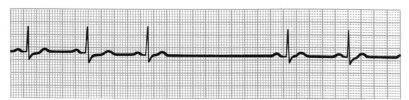

EKG characteristics. PP interval that's not a multiple of the sinus rhythm (an escape beat usually terminates this pause); and dropped

Continued on page 118

Dysrhythmias

Specific dysrhythmias—*continued*

P waves. In complete arrest, no P waves appear.

Clinical implications. Sinus arrest occurs when the SA node fails to generate an impulse. Possible causes include degenerative heart disease, MI, digitalis toxicity, and factors that increase vagal tone.

Interventions. If the patient develops symptomatic bradycardia, the doctor treats this finding and the underlying cause.

Wandering pacemaker

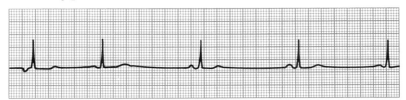

EKG characteristics. Variable rate, irregular PP interval, changeable P-wave configuration (the P wave may be inverted or absent), and variable PR intervals. QRS complexes usually remain normal.

Clinical implications. This dysrhythmia results when the dominant pacemaker shifts from the SA node to other atrial sites, or possibly to AV junctional tissue. Usually transient, wandering pacemaker may be hard to diagnose; the patient may have an irregular pulse while remaining unaware of any problem.

Probably caused by increased vagal tone, wandering pacemaker may appear in athletes, the elderly, and children. When prolonged, it may indicate underlying heart disease.

Interventions. If the patient develops bradycardia, the doctor treats this finding.

Sick sinus syndrome (SSS)

In this dysrhythmia, you'll find alternating tachycardia and bradycardia, interrupted by a long sinus pause. You may also see SA or AV block; sinus bradycardia; or chronic, slow atrial fibrillation.

The term *sick sinus syndrome* applies to rapid-and-slow supraventricular dysrhythmias that cause syncope episodes; it's also called the *Stokes-Adams* or *brady-tachy syndrome.* In addition to syncope, signs and symptoms (which may be episodic and transient) include such subtle changes as forgetfulness and fatigue.

Most common among the elderly, SSS is usually associated with atherosclerosis rather than an acute disorder. Other possible causes include SA node trauma, neuromuscular disorder, inferior- or lateral-wall MI, myocardial ischemia, and rheumatic fever or other inflammatory heart disease.

When an acute disorder causes SSS, the patient usually requires only temporary pacemaker support until the underlying disorder

Dysrhythmias

resolves. When the dysrhythmia's chronic, the doctor may order digitalis or propranolol to manage ventricular response to the tachydysrhythmia; a pacemaker to maintain heart rate and ensure adequate cardiac output; or both.

Atrial dysrhythmias

Premature atrial contraction (PAC)

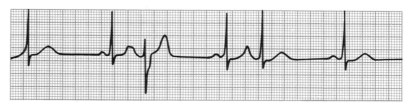

EKG characteristics. Premature and abnormal P waves, possibly lost in the previous T wave; PR intervals longer or shorter than normal; and normal QRS complexes, unless the patient has delayed or absent ventricular conduction. If the impulse arrives in the ventricles during their absolute refractory stage, no QRS complex follows the P wave (known as a nonconducted PAC).

Clinical implications. Expect an irregular pulse; the patient may also complain of palpitations. PACs frequently occur in patients with coronary and valvular heart disease, although PACs may also result from stress, fatigue, or coffee or tobacco ingestion. Drugs that prolong the SA node's absolute refractory period, such as digitalis, quinidine, and procainimide, may increase the incidence of PACs.

Interventions. Most patients don't require treatment. For frequent PACs or those that cause sustained tachycardia, the doctor may order a drug that prolongs atrial refractoriness, such as digitalis, verapamil, or propranolol.

Atrial tachycardia

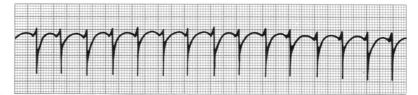

These dysrhythmias usually result from AV nodal reentry or enhanced automaticity of an ectopic focus. Enhanced automaticity probably causes atrial tachycardia with block and multifocal atrial tachycardia (MAT); an AV nodal reentry mechanism probably leads to paroxysmal atrial tachycardia (PAT, also known as paroxysmal supraventricular tachycardia, or PSVT). (See page 123 for more information on SVTs.)

EKG characteristics. Three or more successive atrial ectopic beats occurring at a rate between 160 and 220 beats/minute; upright P wave, or a P wave that's lost in the previous T wave; and normal QRS complexes (in most cases). In MAT, ectopic P-wave configurations vary. Atrial rate varies from 100 to 150 beats/minute. PR and PP intervals also vary.

Atrial overdrive pacing

To halt atrial tachycardia, the doctor may perform atrial overdrive pacing (also called rapid atrial pacing).

By pacing the atria at a rate slightly higher than the patient's intrinsic atrial rate, this technique interferes with the conduction circuit, rendering part of it refractory to the reentrant impulse. This interrupts the established pathway and stops the tachycardia, permitting the sinus node to resume its natural pacemaking role.

In some cases, the doctor may choose a slightly different method, pacing with much faster bursts or pacing prematurely at a critical time in the conduction cycle.

Continued on page 120

Dysrhythmias

Carotid sinus massage

This technique, usually done by the doctor, stimulates the vagus nerve, which in turn inhibits SA node firing and slows AV node conduction. Carotid sinus massage may halt certain supraventricular tachycardias (SVTs), and helps differentiate dysrhythmias.

However, before using carotid sinus massage, the doctor will carefully weigh the possible risks involved: for example, decreased heart rate and vasodilation, possibly leading to cerebral hypotension, and compromised cerebral circulation. This method may also cause cardiac asystole and ventricular dysrhythmias.

Synchronized cardioversion

A patient whose dysrhythmia causes low cardiac output and hypotension may be a candidate for synchronized cardioversion. This technique, which can be done electively or in an emergency, uses a cardioverter (defibrillator). The procedure resembles defibrillation, with one exception: the patient's EKG R wave must be synchronized with the cardioverter (during the R wave, the atria respond best to stimulation, and the ventricles respond least). The doctor depresses the firing buttons, and the cardioverter discharges energy (usually 50 to 200 watt-seconds) when it senses the next R wave.

Important: Synchronized cardioversion should never be used to treat ventricular fibrillation or dysrhythmias stemming from digitalis toxicity.

Specific dysrhythmias—*continued*

Clinical implications. Although seen in patients with normal hearts, atrial tachycardia usually arises in conjunction with a primary cardiac problem (for example, MI, congenital heart disease, cardiomyopathy, or Wolff-Parkinson-White syndrome) or a secondary cardiac problem (such as hyperthyroidism, cor pulmonale, or systemic hypertension). However, digitalis toxicity most frequently precipitates atrial tachycardia. Atrial tachycardia with a persistent rhythm, rapid ventricular rate, or both, may lead to hemodynamic changes; signs and symptoms range from mild palpitations to cardiovascular and pulmonary collapse.

MAT occurs almost exclusively in patients with chronic pulmonary disease, probably from atrial distention secondary to elevated pulmonary pressures.

Interventions. The doctor treats atrial tachycardia according to the severity of the patient's signs and symptoms (although he'll aim treatment of MAT at the underlying disease). In an emergency, vagotonic maneuvers such as the Valsalva maneuver, carotid sinus massage, or synchronized cardioversion may successfully terminate the dysrhythmia or increase the AV block. Overdrive pacing may also end the dysrhythmia. The doctor may order such drugs as digitalis, propranolol, edrophonium, or verapamil.

Atrial flutter

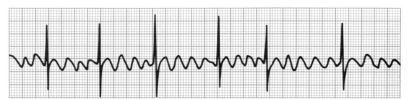

EKG characteristics. Sawtoothed flutter (or F) waves ranging from 220 to 350 beats/minute; variable or constant ratio of atrial to ventricular contractions; and usually normal QRS complexes.

Clinical implications. Atrial flutter may result from prolonged atrial conduction time. It may occur in patients with:
• acute or chronic cardiac disease
• inferior-wall MI (as a transient complication)
• mitral or tricuspid valve disease
• cor pulmonale
• intracardiac infective processes.

Atrial flutter's dangers depend on its ventricular rate. When the dysrhythmia's secondary to an underlying cardiac disorder, even a slight rate increase could compromise ventricular filling and coronary artery blood flow long enough to cause cardiac, cerebral, or peripheral vascular effects (such as syncope, angina, congestive heart failure, pulmonary edema, or hypotension).

Carotid sinus massage can help distinguish atrial flutter from other supraventricular tachycardias. This maneuver usually slows a rapid ventricular response and permits visualization of flutter waves on EKG.

Interventions. A patient with atrial flutter that's accompanied by a rapid ventricular response and reduced cardiac output requires

Dysrhythmias

Understanding Ashman's phenomenon

Ashman's phenomenon—phasic aberrant interventricular conduction of a supraventricular beat—may accompany atrial fibrillation. The abnormal conduction relates to changes in refractory period duration. For example, when a short cycle follows a long cycle, a premature beat may arrive while some tissue remains refractory, thus conducting the impulse abnormally. Such aberrancy may continue for several cycles. EKG characteristics of Ashman's phenomenon include:
● normal initial QRS deflection
● right bundle branch block (RBBB) pattern
● irregular coupling interval of premature beats
● no compensatory pause after the aberrant beat.

Ashman's phenomenon, although a physiologic process, may be misdiagnosed as pathologic ectopic ventricular beats and treated inappropriately with antiarrhythmic drugs.

immediate intervention with synchronized cardioversion or such drugs as digitalis or verapamil. If time and the patient's condition permit, the doctor may use atrial overdrive pacing. Like cardioversion, overdrive pacing stimulates part of the myocardium to depolarize, interrupting circus movement. (See *Atrial overdrive pacing* on page 119 to learn more about this technique.)

For atrial flutter caused by other factors, such as mitral valve disease, the doctor also treats the underlying cause.

Atrial fibrillation

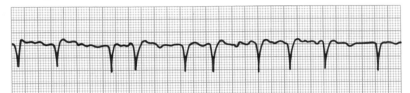

EKG characteristics. Absent P waves; irregular ventricular response (RR interval); and chaotic fibrillatory (f) waves, indicating atrial tetanization from rapid atrial depolarizations (400 to 600 beats/minute). The rhythm's called *coarse* atrial fibrillation when waves appear pronounced, *fine* fibrillation when waves show less marked deflection. The atrial rate greatly exceeds the ventricular rate, because most impulses aren't conducted through the AV junction.

Clinical implications. Atrial fibrillation commonly accompanies rheumatic heart disease, cardiac valve disorders, hypertension, ischemic heart disease, cardiomyopathy, CAD, and thyrotoxicosis. It can also occur with chronic obstructive pulmonary disease (COPD), constrictive pericarditis, or congestive heart failure, and may follow an MI. Other possible causes include exercise and use of certain drugs.

This chaotic atrial rhythm, caused by multiple mechanisms, eliminates the contribution that atrial contraction normally makes to ventricular filling (about 20% to 30% of normal end-diastolic volume). Besides these hemodynamic changes, atrial fibrillation poses danger from possible development of mural thrombi in the fibrillating atria, especially when the dysrhythmia persists.

When assessing a patient with atrial fibrillation, keep in mind that radial pulse rates may be inaccurate, because weaker contractions won't produce a palpable pulse. If your patient has an irregular radial pulse, check his apical pulse.

Interventions. Treatment aims to first control the ventricular response, then produce a normal sinus rhythm. The methods chosen depend on the patient's condition. A hemodynamically unstable patient requires immediate synchronized cardioversion. In an alert patient, the Valsalva maneuver or carotid sinus massage may successfully reduce the ventricular response. (However, don't use these techniques for a patient with chronic atrial fibrillation.)

To increase AV node refractoriness, the doctor may order digitalis, verapamil, or propranolol. Other options include such drugs as quinidine or procainamide to prolong atrial refractoriness, which gives the SA node a chance to resume its role as dominant pacemaker.

To prevent atrial fibrillation from recurring, the doctor treats the

Continued on page 122

Dysrhythmias

Specific dysrhythmias—*continued*

underlying cause. For example, he may surgically correct a valvular disorder or treat congestive heart failure aggressively.

Junctional dysrhythmias

Junctional rhythm

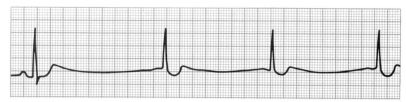

EKG characteristics. Slow, regular rhythm of 40 to 60 beats/minute; normal QRS complexes; and a P wave preceding the QRS complex, with a shortened PR interval, if the junctional impulse conducts antegradely to the ventricles. With retrograde conduction to the atria, the P wave follows the QRS complex or takes an inverted shape. If conduction occurs both antegradely and retrogradely, expect an absent or buried P wave. *Important:* A junctional escape beat appears late (after the next expected beat would normally occur), differentiating it from a premature or early beat.

Clinical implications. Both a junctional escape beat (a single junctional beat) and junctional rhythm (junctional beats that continue for a prolonged time) serve as safety mechanisms, protecting the heart from standstill by "escaping" after suppression of a higher pacemaker site.

If the patient can't tolerate the hemodynamic changes caused by a junctional rhythm, he may experience signs and symptoms of reduced cardiac output.

Interventions. The doctor probably won't treat an asymptomatic patient. But a patient with signs and symptoms requires therapy that increases the sinus or junctional rate, such as atropine; or that supports the ventricular rate, such as a temporary pacemaker. The doctor directs long-term management toward correcting the primary dysrhythmia. *Remember, junctional escape beats serve as safety features; never try to suppress them.*

Premature junctional contraction (PJC)

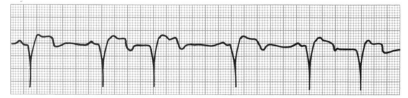

EKG characteristics. Inverted (or otherwise abnormally shaped) P wave before or after the QRS complex; or a P wave hidden in the QRS complex. If a normally shaped P wave appears, expect a shorter-than-normal PR interval. The QRS complex usually has a normal configuration and duration. PJCs appear before the next normally expected complex.

A noncompensatory pause reflecting retrograde conduction to the atria usually accompanies PJCs. (Because PJCs share some features with PACs, take care not to confuse the two dysrhythmias.)

Dysrhythmias

Clinical implications. PJCs commonly result from digitalis toxicity, which enhances automaticity.

Interventions. Most patients don't require treatment. However, if PJCs cause signs or symptoms, the doctor treats the underlying cause.

Junctional tachycardias

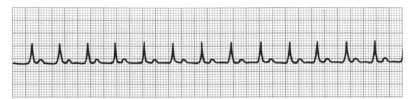

EKG characteristics. In *accelerated junctional rhythm*, a rate between 60 and 100 beats/minute (higher than the inherent rate of junctional tissue); in *junctional tachycardia*, a rate between 100 and 250 beats/minute. Expect a PQRS complex similar to that seen in junctional rhythm. An accelerated rhythm usually has a gradual onset, while junctional tachycardia generally begins and ends abruptly.

Clinical implications. Although most junctional tachycardias stem from the same factors that cause atrial tachycardia, they're more frequently associated with digitalis toxicity.

Interventions. Most patients with accelerated junctional rhythm don't have signs or symptoms, and require no treatment if the ventricular rate's acceptable. Junctional tachycardia, in contrast, may reduce cardiac output, especially at faster rates. The doctor may order cardioversion, vagotonic maneuvers, or therapy with digitalis, propranolol, verapamil, or edrophonium.

Supraventricular tachycardias (SVTs)

The term *supraventricular tachycardia* refers to any tachydysrhythmia that originates above the His bundle bifurcation. The term SVT may be used when the tachycardia type can't be clearly identified. For convenience, we'll categorize SVTs as follows:
• those arising from an ectopic focus (for example, atrial tachycardia with block, multifocal atrial tachycardia, and junctional tachycardia). A common cause: enhanced automaticity from digitalis toxicity.
• those arising from an AV nodal reentry mechanism (also called PSVTs). This group also includes PATs and paroxysmal junctional tachycardias [PJTs]. The initial ectopic beat arises in the atria or junction, resulting in an AV nodal reentry tachycardia.

SVTs can be more easily recognized when QRS complexes resemble those of sinus-conducted beats, revealing a focus above the His bundle bifurcation. In some cases, SVT conduction through the ventricles (usually the right bundle branch) may be partially blocked. This phenomenon, known as aberrant ventricular conduction, causes an abnormal QRS complex (see page 130 for more on aberrant conduction).

Preexcitation syndromes

Preexcitation, also known as accelerated conduction, refers to abnormal conduction of an atrial impulse to the ventricles, resulting in early ventricular depolarization. This occurs via a pathway outside the normal AV nodal-His bundle-Purkinje conduction pathway.

Continued on page 124

Dysrhythmias

Specific dysrhythmias—*continued*

Normally, the annulus fibrosus (a ring of nonconducting tissue) separates the atria and the ventricles. Only the AV node and His bundle junction interrupt this ring. In preexcitation, however, a congenital anomolous pathway bridges the annulus fibrosus, connecting the atria to the ventricles at a different location. This pathway conducts impulses from the atria to the ventricles more quickly than does the AV-nodal pathway, causing preexcitation. As a result, a portion of the ventricles depolarizes prematurely.

Wolff-Parkinson-White (WPW) syndrome. The most common preexcitation syndrome, WPW occurs when an atrial bypass tract outside the AV junction (probably the Kent bundles) connects the atria and the ventricles. This tract can conduct impulses either antegradely to the ventricles or retrogradely to the atria. With retrograde conduction, a reentrant circuit can arise.

On EKG, expect to see a PR interval less than 0.12 second and a QRS complex greater than 0.12 second; the beginning of the QRS complex may be slurred from premature partial ventricular depolarization via the bypass tract. This slurring produces a delta wave—the hallmark of WPW.

You may also find ST-segment and T-wave changes in the direction opposite to the QRS complex and SVTs with a ventricular rate as fast as 300 beats/minute. The fast rate may result from circus reentry, which sustains the tachycardia. Circus movement interruption may occur when the refractoriness or conduction time of either pathway changes (spontaneously or through medical intervention). Atrial fibrillation may accompany WPW if the ventricular response rate exceeds 180 beats/minute.

WPW occurs most commonly in young children or adults age 20 to 35. The patient may complain of sudden chest pain, shortness of breath, and palpitations. If WPW causes a rapid ventricular response, cardiovascular collapse can ensue.

WPW with a fast ventricular response requires quick intervention. To slow the tachycardia, the doctor may perform vagotonic maneuvers or order drugs (such as propranolol, quinidine, procainamide, verapamil, or lidocaine) to increase the absolute refractory period of the AV node or bypass tract. He may perform cardioversion if other interventions fail.

In less urgent situations, treatment depends on the patient's signs and symptoms. EP studies can help pinpoint the bypass tract's location and determine treatment when WPW causes an extremely rapid ventricular rate. Management consists of drug therapy or possibly surgical ablation (usually cryosurgery).

Lown-Ganong-Levin (LGL) syndrome. The second major preexcitation syndrome, LGL occurs less commonly than WPW. The bypass tract responsible for the reentrant tachycardia (probably the James bundle) connects the atrium to the AV node's lower portion or the bundle of His.

On EKG, check for an abnormally short but constant PR interval (because the SA node impulse travels to the bundle of His more quickly by the bypass tract), normal P waves, and normal QRS complexes.

Dysrhythmias

LGL produces a short PR interval, possibly attributable to an ectopic atrial pacemaker. However, the PR interval remains constant, and P-wave configuration remains normal.

The doctor treats LPL as he treats WPW.

Atrioventricular heart block (AV block)

Any delay or interruption in impulse conduction constitutes heart block. In AV block, the interruption occurs between the atria and ventricles, preventing the impulse from reaching the ventricles when it should. Causes include ischemic or rheumatic heart disease, MI, myocarditis, congenital heart defects, degenerative heart disease, hypothyroidism, hypoxia, digitalis toxicity, and hyperkalemia.

AV block's classified by degree as follows.

First-degree AV block

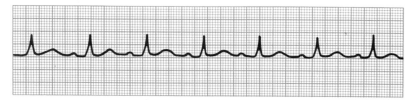

EKG characteristics. Prolonged but constant PR interval greater than 0.20 second.

Clinical implications. This block, which delays all supraventricular impulses through the conduction system, usually occurs transiently. It may appear in healthy persons; or it can result from drug therapy (such as quinidine, pronestyl, propranolol, or digitalis), rheumatic fever, or a chronic degenerative disease of the conduction system.

Interventions. Most patients need no treatment. But if a patient develops symptomatic bradycardia, the doctor may order atropine.

Second-degree AV block

This condition blocks one or more—but not all—supraventricular impulses. Second degree block occurs in two types: Type I (Wenckebach or Mobitz I) and Type II (Mobitz II).

● *Type I second-degree AV block (Wenckebach or Mobitz I)*

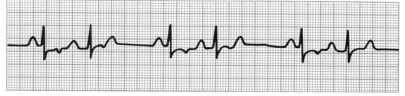

EKG characteristics. Constant PP intervals; progressively lengthening PR intervals; progressively shortening RR intervals, until a P wave appears without a QRS complex (dropped beat). The next conducted beat has a short PR interval and the QRS complex usually appears normal.

Group beating ("the footprints of Wenckebach") usually distinguishes this dysrhythmia. In each group, the first PR interval's only slightly prolonged, with the largest increment falling between the first and second intervals. The RR interval encompassing the dropped beat measures less than twice the shortest cycle.

Continued on page 126

Dysrhythmias

High-grade AV block

A high-grade, or advanced, AV block occurs when two or more consecutive supraventricular impulses fail to conduct; the atrial rate generally remains below 135 beats/minute. This pattern occurs when the conduction system's prolonged refractoriness permits latent pacemaker discharge.

High-grade AV block frequently triggers escape rhythms. Because it reduces heart rate, it may also decrease cardiac output, possibly leading to Stokes-Adams syncope. High-grade AV block may progress to third-degree block.

Specific dysrhythmias—*continued*

Clinical implications. Type I block, often transient, occurs with rheumatic fever, use of such drugs as digitalis and propranolol, and inferior-wall MI. After the cause has been resolved or eliminated, this block disappears.

Interventions. Most patients need no treatment.

- *Type II second-degree AV block (Mobitz II)*

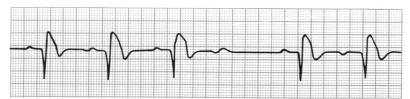

EKG characteristics. Constant PP and PR intervals and sudden dropped beat. The interval containing the nonconducted P wave equals two normal PP intervals. The QRS complex may be prolonged.

Clinical implications. This block usually occurs at or below the bundle of His. Usually chronic, it can accompany organic heart disease or appear after acute anterior-wall MI. It may progress to a higher block.

Interventions. Treatment depends on the patient's symptoms. If the patient's hypotensive, the doctor will probably order isoproterenol to maintain cardiac output. Long-term management requires pacemaker insertion to prevent ventricular standstill.

Third-degree AV block (complete heart block [CHB]).

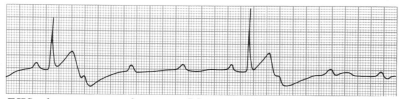

EKG characteristics. Constant PP intervals, with no relationship between the P wave and QRS complexes. QRS configuration depends on where the ventricular beat originates. Ventricular rate's usually less than 45 beats/minute.

Clinical implications. This condition, which leads to complete blockage of all supraventricular impulses to the ventricles, can be acute or chronic. When acute, it may be associated with severe digitalis toxicity, or inferior-wall or anterior wall MI.

Chronic CHB most frequently stems from bilateral bundle branch block resulting from widespread His-Purkinje system changes. Other causes include Lev's disease (fibrosis and calcification that spreads from such cardiac structures as the valves and septum to the conductive tissue) and Lenegre's disease (fibrosis of the conductive tissue).

Signs and symptoms depend on the stability of the escape rhythm and the patient's response to ventricular rate decreases.

Interventions. Immediate therapy aims to support, and then maintain, a stable ventricular rhythm. If the patient has adequate cardiac output, he may not need treatment. But if his cardiac output's inadequate—or if his condition will likely deteriorate—the doctor

Dysrhythmias

may order atropine or isoproterenol, followed by pacemaker insertion. *Note:* Avoid giving isoproterenol to a CHB patient who's had an acute MI.

Bundle branch blocks

These blocks, which involve impulse conduction disorders in a particular segment of the intraventricular conduction system, include right and left bundle branch blocks and hemiblocks.

Frequently associated with MI, such blocks may also accompany valvular disease, congenital anomalies, ventricular hypertrophy, and atherosclerosis of the conduction system.

Bundle branch blocks typically produce prolonged QRS complexes, the result of decreased conduction velocity. Characteristics of *complete* bundle branch block (of either branch) include QRS duration greater than 0.12 second. QRS duration between 0.10 and 0.12 second usually indicates *incomplete* bundle branch block. You'll also see a late intrinsicoid deflection.

Right bundle branch block   Left bundle branch block

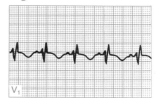 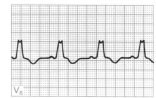

Right bundle branch block (RBBB)
This dysrhythmia doesn't interfere with the initial left-to-right direction of the ventricular depolarizing force. A late intrinsicoid deflection in leads V_1 and V_2 results from late activation of the right ventricle, as depolarizing forces spread through the septum from the left ventricle. The ventricular complexes in RBBB may take one of the following shapes: RSR[1], RR[1], or an M-shaped pattern that usually appears in leads V_1 and V_2.

In leads V_5 and V_6, the initial Q wave and the intrinsicoid deflection remain normal. However, expect a widened S wave from delayed right ventricular activation. RBBB may occur in normal or diseased hearts.

Left bundle branch block (LBBB)
This block disrupts normal left-to-right ventricular activation pattern. Instead, the depolarizing impulse travels down the right bundle from right to left, spreading to the left ventricle through the interventricular septum.

Leads V_5 and V_6 give the best evidence of LBBB. The initial Q waves normally seen in those leads don't appear; the main QRS deflection appears wide and notched, with a late intrinsicoid deflection. In leads V_1 and V_2, look for a widened S wave.

Hemiblock
This can occur in either fascicle of the left bundle. Left anterior hemiblock (LAH) refers to block in the anterosuperior fascicle; left posterior hemiblock (LPH) refers to a block of the posteroinferior fascicle. Blockage of either left bundle division shifts the terminal portion of the QRS complex in the direction of the blocked division, resulting in axis deviation.

Continued on page 128

Dysrhythmias

Specific dysrhythmias—*continued*

In LAH, EKG features include a small Q wave in lead I and an RS pattern in lead III. The QRS complex may appear normal. By itself, LAH isn't significant; however, it's frequently associated with RBBB or an anterior MI.

In LPH, EKG characteristics include small R and deep S waves in lead I, and small Q and tall R waves in lead III. LPH alone doesn't require treatment. However, if RBBB accompanies this pattern, stay alert for complete heart block.

Ventricular dysrhythmias

Premature ventricular contraction (PVC)

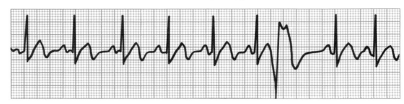

EKG characteristics. Wide (greater than 0.12 second), bizarre QRS complexes because the impulse arises from the ventricle; absent P waves; slow rate; usually regular rhythm; and T waves in the opposite direction of the wide QRS complex. A long horizontal baseline called a compensatory pause generally follows the T wave. However, not all PVCs have compensatory pauses. (Those that don't are called interpolated PVCs). A compensatory pause exists if the PP interval encompassing the PVC has twice the duration of a normal sinus beat's PP interval.

Clinical implications. Among the most common dysrhythmias, PVCs can arise in both healthy and diseased hearts. The mechanism producing these beats (also called ventricular extrasystolic beats) remains unclear, but the following factors may contribute:
- Digitalis toxicity
- Hypokalemia
- Hypocalcemia
- Caffeine, tobacco, and alcohol ingestion
- Sympathomimetic drugs (for example, epinephrine and isoproterenol)
- Myocardial irritation by pacemaker electrodes
- Exercise.

PVCs on a single rhythm strip that all look alike (for instance, all having an upward positive deflection or downward negative deflection) go by the name *unifocal PVCs*. These complexes arise from the same ectopic focus. The term *multifocal PVCs* refers to PVCs that look different from one another. For example, one might be wider with a downward deflection, another slightly thinner with an upward deflection. Such complexes indicate impulse generation from two different ventricular sites, a more ominous sign.

Benign PVCs, occurring in the absence of heart disease or arising infrequently in an asymptomatic patient, require no treatment. But the following PVC patterns require special attention:
- two or more PVCs in a row. (Two successive PVCs are called a couplet, or pair; three or more, a salvo or run of ventricular tachycardia.)

Identifying idioventricular rhythm

If the cells of the His-Purkinje system take over as the heart's pacemaker, an idioventricular rhythm results. This occurs when the SA or AV node fails or when blockage prevents supraventricular impulses from entering the ventricles (for instance, from MI or digitalis toxicity).

An idioventricular rhythm has wide, bizarre QRS complexes and absent P waves. Its rate ranges from 20 to 40 beats/minute and its rhythm usually remains regular.

If only one ventricular beat appears, consider this a ventricular escape beat rather than idioventricular rhythm. Considered a safety mechanism, a ventricular escape beat occurs late in the cycle and shouldn't be suppressed.

Occasionally, you may see an EKG pattern with all the characteristics of idioventricular rhythm, but with a rate between 50 and 100 beats/minute. This may be an accelerated idioventricular rhythm resulting from slowed conduction through the SA node. Take care not to confuse accelerated idioventricular rhythm with a slow ventricular tachycardia. Avoid giving lidocaine. Used to treat tachydysrhythmias, this drug abolishes ventricular function, possibly causing asystole in a patient with idioventricular rhythm.

Notify the doctor and order a stat 12-lead EKG if your patient develops this rhythm, and check the patient's condition. The doctor may insert an atrial pacemaker and possibly also order atropine to counter the bradycardia.

Dysrhythmias

Other ventricular tachycardias

Ventricular tachycardia can take various forms. Ventricular flutter has an extremely rapid rate (200 to 400 beats/minute) and a regular up-and-down sweeping form with no discernible P or T waves. This potentially fatal dysrhythmia halts breathing and causes an absent palpable pulse. Intervention includes immediate defibrillation or CPR if a defibrillator's not available.

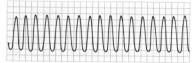
Ventricular flutter

Torsades de Pointes gets its name from its EKG configuration: the QRS polarity seems to spiral around the isoelectric line. Its rate ranges from 200 to 240 beats/minute.

The R-on-T phenomenon can trigger Torsades. Although sinus rhythm sometimes resumes spontaneously, Torsades may degenerate into ventricular fibrillation. Any condition causing a prolonged QT interval can also cause Torsades.

The patient will have signs and symptoms similar to those of ventricular tachycardia. However, treatment differs from standard ventricular tachycardia therapy. Most important, if misdiagnosed as another dysrhythmia, Torsades may not respond to—or may worsen from—drugs such as quinidine, lidocaine, or tocainide.

The doctor will generally stabilize Torsades with mechanical pacing, or order antiarrhythmics, such as isoproterenol (the drug of choice), bretylium, propanolol, or phenytoin.

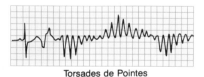
Torsades de Pointes

- bigeminy (when every other beat's a PVC) or trigeminy (when every third beat's a PVC)
- multifocal PVCs
- more than six PVCs per minute
- R-on-T phenomenon. This danger sign appears when the PVC occurs so prematurely that it falls on the preceding beat's T wave. The T-wave peak represents the cell's relative refractory (or vulnerable) period. A PVC that occurs then, before cells fully repolarize, can cause ventricular tachycardia or fibrillation. If you see this pattern on your patient's EKG, check his condition and notify the doctor immediately.

PVCs may increase atrial diastolic filling time during the compensatory pause, making the heart work harder to eject the additional blood on the next sinus beat. They also decrease cardiac output. Thus, a PVC's clinical significance hinges on how well the ventricle functions and how long the dysrhythmia lasts. In an ischemic or damaged heart, PVCs will more likely develop into ventricular tachycardia, flutter, or fibrillation than in a healthy heart.

Interventions. The doctor may order oxygen, potassium, or antiarrhythmic drugs such as lidocaine. Treatment will also depend on the cause. If the patient has bradycardia, the doctor may order atropine to raise the heart rate instead of an antiarrhythmic. The reason: bradycardia can cause myocardial irritation and stimulate PVCs. By treating bradycardia, the doctor may eliminate PVCs without using an antiarrhythmic. If the patient has a pacemaker, the doctor may reposition the electrodes—another possible source of myocardial irritation. Direct your nursing interventions toward reducing the heart's work load and, thus, decreasing myocardial oxygen needs.

Ventricular tachycardia

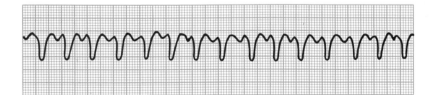

EKG characteristics. Wide, bizarre QRS complexes; regular rhythm; fast rate (100 to 180 beats/minute); absent P waves; and T waves pointing in the direction opposite to QRS complexes.

Clinical implications. Myocardial irritability generally causes this life-threatening dysrhythmia. Patients at risk for ventricular tachycardia include those with a history of MI, CAD, rheumatic heart disease, mitral valve prolapse, or cardiomyopathy. This dysrhythmia can lead to ventricular fibrillation and thus warrants emergency intervention. A patient whose cardiac output drops precipitously from the rapid ventricular rate risks cardiovascular collapse.

Interventions. If you observe signs of ventricular tachycardia on EKG, immediately check the patient's condition and notify the doctor. If the patient's alert, expect to give an antiarrhythmic such as lidocaine, as ordered. But if the patient suffers cardiovascular collapse and loses consciousness, prepare for defibrillation. Perform CPR until a defibrillator's available.

Continued on page 130

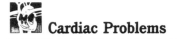

Dysrhythmias

Aberrant ventricular conduction

This dysrhythmia reflects temporary abnormal intraventricular conduction of supraventricular impulses. Because it mimics ventricular ectopic beats, it may be hard to identify. But remember, an aberrant beat originates from an atrial stimulus that's conducted abnormally through the ventricles; a ventricular ectopic beat originates from a ventricular impulse.

Expect an aberrant beat to have a wide QRS complex (greater than 0.12 second) preceded by an ectopic P wave. Lack of a full compensatory pause after the questionable beat suggests aberrancy.

If your patient has a history of bundle branch block, compare a previous 12-lead EKG strip showing this block with the strip in question. If the QRS complexes look similar, suspect aberrancy.

To differentiate ventricular from supraventricular aberrant tachycardia, try using the Valsalva manuever. If your patient's heart rate slows while he bears down, suspect tachycardia of supraventricular origin. (Vagal stimulation from the maneuver rarely affects ventricular impulses.)

If the patient's on a cardiac monitor, the doctor may use carotid massage, another form of vagal stimulation, to identify the tachycardia. Massage will slow supraventricular (but not ventricular) tachycardia. (*Note:* Carotid massage can compromise cerebral perfusion if the patient has carotid artery bruits.)

Specific dysrhythmias—*continued*
Ventricular fibrillation

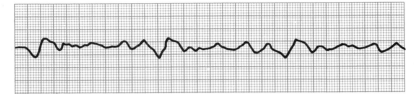

EKG characteristics. Chaotic and rapid ventricular rhythm with unidentifiable QRS complexes. Large waves indicate *coarse fibrillation*, small waves, *fine fibrillation*.

Clinical implications. Ventricular fibrillation halts cardiac output by causing the ventricles to quiver rather than contract. The patient lacks a pulse, audible heart sounds, and respirations.

Interventions. Begin CPR and prepare for defibrillation as soon as possible—it's the only effective treatment. The chance for successful defibrillation improves with administration of I.V. agents such as epinephrine, lidocaine, procainamide, or bretylium. (For more information on defibrillation and cardiac arrest, see Chapter 9.)

Self Test

1. Myocardial cells can't respond to a stimulus during the:
a. absolute refractory period   **b.** relative refractory period   **c.** vulnerable period   **d.** excitability period

2. A tall, tented T wave may indicate:
a. hypokalemia   **b.** hyperkalemia   **c.** hypocalcemia   **d.** hypercalcemia

3. When using lead II cardiac monitoring, place the positive electrode:
a. at the fourth intercostal space, at the right sternal border   **b.** on the left shoulder, below the clavicular hollow   **c.** on the right shoulder, below the clavicular hollow   **d.** on the left side of the chest at the lowest palpable rib, along the midclavicular line

4. Mr. Derrickson, a cardiac care unit patient, has an artificial ventricular demand pacemaker. On his cardiac monitor, you note pacemaker spikes not followed by QRS complexes. You suspect:
a. failure to pace   **b.** failure to sense   **c.** failure to capture   **d.** none of the above

5. Nursing interventions for Mr. Derrickson may include:
a. placing a magnet over the pacemaker   **b.** adjusting the sensitivity dial   **c.** replacing the pacemaker battery   **d.** turning him on his left side

6. Premature ventricular contractions have all of the following characteristics, except:
a. a compensatory pause after the premature beat (usually)   **b.** a T wave in the direction opposite the QRS complex   **c.** a P wave before the premature beat   **d.** a wide, bizarre QRS complex

Answers (page number shows where answer appears in text)

1. **a** (page 104)   2. **b** (page 107)   3. **d** (page 107)   4. **c** (page 114)
5. **d** (page 114)   6. **c** (page 128)

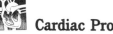

Cardiac Arrest/Cardiac Trauma: Deadly Threats

Mary Cooney wrote the section on cardiac arrest. A staff nurse in the intensive cardiac care unit at Grandview Hospital in Sellersville, Pa., she received her ADN from Middlessex County College, Edison, N.J.

Margaret T. Perrone contributed the sections on cardiac trauma, cough CPR, and the automatic implantable defibrillator. Ms. Perrone, who earned her BSN from the University of Michigan, is a staff nurse at the University of Michigan Hospitals, Ann Arbor.

What causes cardiac arrest

Cause/Precipitated by:

Inadequate blood flow
Pulmonary embolus
Air embolus
Hemorrhage
Thrombus formation

Ineffective cardiac contractility
Heart failure
Cardiac rupture
Myocardial infarction
Cardiac tamponade

Insufficient conduction
Hypokalemia
Hyperkalemia
Electrical shock, mechanical trauma
(cardiac surgery)
Severe acidosis
Hypothermia
Idiopathic dysrhythmia
Cardiac pacemaker dysfunction
Hypoxemia
Myocardial infarction

Adapted from Ellis, P.D. and Billings, D.M. *Cardiopulmonary Resuscitation: Procedures for Basic and Advanced Life Support,* C.V. Mosby Co., 1980, p 20.

Cardiac arrest

When the heart suddenly stops pumping effectively as a result of ventricular fibrillation, ventricular asystole, or electromechanical dissociation, cardiac arrest occurs. Your patient's life could depend on your ability to quickly assess the situation: unless respiration and circulation resume, he'll suffer clinical death. Biological death follows in 4 to 6 minutes when brain cells start to die.

Assessment

Suspect cardiac arrest in any patient who suddenly collapses. Lack of a pulse in major vessels and absent heart sounds clinically confirm cardiac arrest. Even though the patient may continue breathing for a few minutes, he'll quickly grow cyanotic and lose consciousness. An electrocardiogram (EKG) may confirm cardiac arrest and also distinguish the cause of arrest from among the three possibilities mentioned above.

Planning

If your assessment suggests cardiac arrest, start cardiopulmonary resuscitation (CPR) immediately. CPR involves the ABCs of resuscitation: airway, breathing, and circulation. (Follow the latest recommended guidelines of the American Heart Association or the American Red Cross for Basic Life Support [BLS] techniques. To stay current with these guidelines, get certified annually by either organization.) If you work in a hospital, call a cardiac code. Follow hospital policy and procedure for cardiac arrest, and be sure to document your actions.

Intervention

No matter what's caused your patient's cardiac arrest, restore his respiration and circulation, using CPR, as your first priority. An exception: the patient who suffers ventricular fibrillation while being monitored on EKG. In this case, defibrillate at once (if hospital policy allows).

In some cases, resuscitation may fail until the precipitating abnormality of the cardiac arrest (for example, Torsades de Pointes or hypomagnesemia) has been treated. For this reason, try to establish what's caused the arrest, while continuing CPR.

You may also need to begin Advanced Cardiac Life Support (ACLS), which supplements BLS measures. ACLS includes adjunctive breathing and circulation techniques and equipment, cardiac monitoring and dysrhythmia recognition (see Chapter 8), and definitive therapy, which encompasses I.V. infusions, drug therapy, defibrillation, and acid-base analysis.

Adjunctive airway and ventilation measures include oxygen administration, artificial airways (oropharyngeal, nasopharyngeal, and esophageal obturator airways and endotracheal intubation), and bag mask devices (such as the AMBU bag).

Circulatory adjuncts include the cardiac press (a manually operated chest compressor), the automatic chest compressor (which uses compressed gas and performs external cardiac compression and artificial ventilation), and medical antishock trousers (MAST),

Continued on page 134

Cardiac Arrest/Cardiac Trauma

EKG rhythms seen in cardiac arrest

Ventricular fibrillation
Characteristics:
- Ventricular rhythm rapid and chaotic, indicating varying degrees of depolarization and repolarization; QRS complexes not identifiable
- Patient unconscious at onset
- Absent pulses, heart sounds, and blood pressure
- Dilated pupils, rapid development of cyanosis

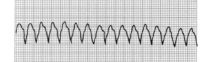

Ventricular asystole (cardiac standstill)
Characteristics:
- Totally absent ventricular electrical activity
- Possible P waves
- Possible severe metabolic deficit or extensive myocardial damage

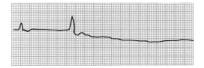

Electromechanical dissociation (EMD) (electrical activity but no pulse)
Characteristics:
- Organized electrical activity without any evidence of effective myocardial contraction
- Possible failure in the calcium transport system (can cause EMD)
- Possible association with profound hypovolemia, cardiac tamponade, myocardial rupture, massive myocardial infarction, or tension pneumothorax

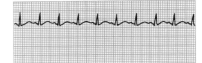

Reviewing code drugs

Drug/Route/Dose	Indications/Effects	Precautions/Warnings
Atropine sulfate *I.V. push:* Yes; administer 0.5 mg over 1 to 2 minutes; can be repeated every 5 minutes; total dose shouldn't exceed 2 mg *Infusion:* Not recommended *Intratracheal:* Yes	• Used for treating excessive vagus-induced bradycardia; first-degree atrioventricular (AV) block, Mobitz I AV block • Increases heart rate • Decreases salivation and respiratory secretions • Decreases smooth muscle spasm	• Lower doses (less than 0.5 mg) may *cause* bradycardia. • Higher doses (more than 2 mg) may cause full vagal blockage. • Contraindicated for glaucoma patients (use isoproterenol instead)
Bretylium tosylate (Bretylol, Bretylate) *I.V. push:* Yes; rapidly administer 5 mg/kg; can be repeated in 15 to 30 minutes to total of 30 mg/kg *Infusion:* Yes; 500 mg diluted to at least 50 ml with 5% D₅W or normal saline solution; infuse at 1 to 2 mg/min	• Used for treating ventricular dysrhythmias that are unresponsive to lidocaine • Positive inotropic effect • Antiarrhythmic effect	• Generally not used to treat PVCs unless other drugs fail • May increase digitalis toxicity • May decrease blood pressure (BP)
Calcium chloride *I.V. push:* Yes; administer 5 to 10 ml of 10% solution at 1 ml/min; can be repeated every 10 minutes *Infusion:* Not generally; can add to D₅W or normal saline; flow rate shouldn't exceed 1.5 mEq/min	• Used for treating asystole and electromechanical dissociation of the heart • Used for treating hyperkalemia • Positive inotropic effect	• Contraindicated in patients with hypercalcemia • Infiltration may produce severe tissue damage. • Use cautiously in patients receiving digoxin; may produce dysrhythmias. • Don't give to patients with high serum phosphate; may produce fatal calcium phosphate deposits in vital organs. • Don't mix with any other medications, especially with alkaline solutions where it will precipitate.
Dobutamine hydrochloride (Dobutrex) *I.V. push:* Not recommended *Infusion:* Yes; reconstitute with D₅W or normal saline solution, then prepare standard dilution; administer 2.5 to 10 mcg/kg/min	• Used for short-term treatment to increase cardiac output • Increases cardiac contractility • May increase urine output	• Don't use with beta-blockers, such as propranolol. • Incompatible with alkaline solutions • Patients with atrial fibrillation should receive digoxin first, or they can develop rapid ventricular response. • Infiltration may produce severe tissue damage.
Dopamine hydrochloride (Intropin) *I.V. push:* Not recommended *Infusion:* Yes; standard dilution; may use with D₅W, dextrose 5% in normal saline solution, or dextrose 5% in ½-normal saline solution; administer 2 to 5 mcg/kg/min, up to 50 mcg/kg/min	• Used for treating cardiogenic shock and other hemodynamic problems, hypotension, and decreased cardiac output • Improves renal perfusion • Increases cardiac output	• Don't use for treating uncorrected tachydysrhythmias or ventricular fibrillation. • May precipitate dysrhythmias • Incompatible with alkaline solutions • Infiltration may produce severe tissue damage. • Solution deteriorates after 24 hours.

Continued

Cardiac Arrest/Cardiac Trauma

Defibrillation: What you should know

Defibrillation can convert life-threatening ventricular fibrillation or ventricular tachycardia to normal cardiac rhythm. The defibrillator consists of a high-voltage power supply, which charges an energy capacitor and two electrode paddles. It delivers an electric shock of several thousand volts, lasting 4 to 12 milliseconds. Most direct-current (DC) defibrillators deliver a maximum of 360 watt-seconds, or joules.

The first defibrillation attempt should range from 200 to 300 watt-seconds for an adult. If unsuccessful, medical workers promptly administer a second shock of the same energy. Open-heart defibrillation requires only 5- to 40-watt-seconds countershock. For infants and children, 2-watt-seconds/kg of body weight should be used for the first attempt; 4-watt-seconds/kg of body weight should be used for the second attempt.

The length of time the patient's been in ventricular fibrillation will influence the outcome of defibrillation. The shorter the fibrillation time, the better his prognosis.

Success also depends on the patient's myocardial condition. Such conditions as hypoxemia, acidosis, hypothermia, electrolyte imbalance, and drug toxicity make the myocardium more resistant to defibrillation.

Electrical resistance of the skin can also prevent successful defibrillation. For proper results, apply a conductive, low-resistance (impedance) paste or gel to the electrode paddles. Be careful not to create a paste path between the paddles.

Important: Be sure to check hospital protocol regarding this procedure.

Reviewing code drugs—*continued*

Drug/Route/Dose	Indications/Effects	Precautions/Warnings
Epinephrine hydrochloride (Adrenalin) *I.V. push:* Yes; administer 5 to 10 ml of 1:10,000 solution (0.5 to 1 mg) over 1 minute *Intracardiac:* Yes; administer 5 ml of 1:10,000 solution (0.5 mg) *Intratracheal:* Yes *Infusion:* Not generally; can mix 2 mg with 500 ml D_5W; administer at 1 to 4 mcg/min	• Used for treating asystole and ventricular fibrillation • A potent sympathomimetic that stimulates both alpha- and beta-receptor cells • Increases cardiac output and systolic blood pressure; relaxes bronchial spasms; mobilizes liver glycogen stores	• Increases intraocular pressure • May exacerbate congestive heart failure, dysrhythmias, angina pectoris, hyperthyroidism, and emphysema • May cause headache, tremors, or palpitations
Isoproterenol hydrochloride (Isuprel) *I.V. push:* Yes; administer 0.02 to 0.04 mg (1 to 2 ml of 1:50,000 solution, which is 1 ml of 1:50,000 diluted with 9 ml of saline *Infusion:* Yes; use standard dilution, administer at 0.5 to 5 mcg/min and titrate as needed	• Used in treating complete heart block and asystole • Functions as a sympathomimetic; affects beta-receptors only, not alpha-receptors	• Don't administer with epinephrine. • Don't mix with barbiturates, sodium bicarbonate, any calcium preparation, or aminophylline.
Lidocaine hydrochloride (Xylocaine) *I.V. push:* Yes; administer 50 to 100 mg; can be repeated every 5 minutes; total dose should not exceed 300 mg in 1-hour period. *Infusion:* Yes; standard dilution, administer at 1 to 4 mg/min *Intratracheal:* Yes	• Used in treating PVCs and ventricular tachycardia • Increases electrical stimulation threshold, especially in ventricular dysrhythmias • Doesn't affect contractility	• Don't mix with sodium bicarbonate. • Don't use if patient has high-grade sinoatrial or AV block. • Discontinue if PR interval or QRS complex widens, or if dysrhythmias become worse • May lead to central nervous system (CNS) toxicity
Procainamide hydrochloride (Pronestyl) *I.V. push:* Yes; administer 500 mg (slow push); can be repeated in 5 minutes; total dose shouldn't exceed 1 g *Infusion:* Yes; infuse at 1 to 4 mg/min	• Used for treating PVCs and ventricular fibrillation when lidocaine is not effective • Depresses the myocardium's response to electrical stimulation and slows conduction	• Can cause precipitous hypotension; don't use for treating second- or third-degree heart block unless a pacemaker's been inserted. • Can cause AV block
Sodium bicarbonate *I.V. push:* Yes; rapidly administer 44.6 mEq in 50 ml D_5W (1 mEq/kg); can be repeated every 10 minutes, depending on blood gases *Infusion:* Not recommended *Intratracheal:* No	• Used in treating cardiac arrest • Facilitates defibrillation by reversing metabolic acidosis	• Don't mix with epinephrine; causes epinephrine degradation. • Don't mix with calcium salts; forms insoluble precipitates.
Verapamil (Isoptin, Calan) *I.V. push:* Yes; administer 5 to 10 mg (0.075 to 0.15 mg/kg) over a minimum of 2 minutes; for older patients, administer over 3 minutes; can be repeated in 30 minutes *Infusion:* For maintenance only—infuse at 0.005 mg/kg/min	• Used in treating supraventricular tachydysrhythmias • Inhibits the influx of calcium ions through the myocardial and vascular smooth muscle cells • Restores normal sinus rhythm in patients with paroxysmal supraventricular tachycardias	• Contraindicated in patients with hypotension, cardiogenic shock, severe congestive heart failure, and second- or third-degree AV block • High doses or administering too rapidly can cause a significant drop in BP.

Cardiac Arrest/Cardiac Trauma

Cardiac arrest—*continued*

(which increase circulating blood volume, and internal cardiac compression).

In the hospital, internal cardiac compression may help a patient with one of the following conditions: an anatomic abnormality (such as chest deformity or emphysema); a penetrating chest trauma; cardiac tamponade; or a crush chest injury. It may also benefit the patient who's in surgery with his chest already opened.

I.V. infusions, part of ACLS' definitive therapy, permit administration of medications and fluids.

In determining a patient's acid-base status, keep in mind that acidosis that occurs during cardiopulmonary arrest usually results from ventilatory failure, as the blood retains carbon dioxide and accumulates lactic and pyruvic acid from anaerobic metabolism. Acidosis suppresses Purkinje fiber depolarization, heightens susceptibility to ventricular fibrillation, diminishes ventricular contractile force, and reduces the heart's responsiveness to catecholamines. Management generally involves pulmonary ventilation and administration of sodium bicarbonate, as determined by arterial blood gas (ABG) analysis.

Also a part of definitive therapy, medications can help reverse hypoxia and metabolic acidosis, increase perfusion pressure during chest compression, spur spontaneous or more forceful myocardial contraction, increase heart rate, and suppress ventricular ectopic

---

Cough CPR: New weapon against ventricular dysrhythmias

A simple reflex mechanism—the cough—may help convert lethal ventricular dysrhythmias to normal sinus rhythm.

The cough has been used mainly in the cardiac catherization laboratory. But researchers have found that continuous, forced coughing spurts, 1 to 3 seconds apart, and just before or at the onset of ventricular tachycardia or fibrillation, can help the patient maintain consciousness for up to 30 seconds.

Cough CPR gives laboratory personnel time to prepare for defibrillation while the patient remains conscious, maintaining blood perfusion to his brain. And the patient can perform it on his own, in any position and on any surface.

How does cough CPR work? By closing the epiglottis and strongly contracting the respiratory muscles, it greatly increases intrathoracic pressure. The compressive force of such a pressure increase propels blood forward (as shown in the illustrations at right). Researchers be-

lieve increased coronary perfusion, which decreases myocardial ischemia, also occurs during cough CPR, from increased aortic pressure and reflex coronary vasodilation secondary to baroreceptor activation.

Cough CPR's other advantages include its ready availability and immediate effectiveness. The method also enables the patient to remain conscious in the face of a lethal dysrhythmia while personnel prepare other interventions. And because the patient takes a breath between each cough, he maintains cardiac and pulmonary function.

All cough CPR candidates must be capable of sustaining an adequate cough. (Many patients have long but ineffective coughing spells.)

If your patient's scheduled for cardiac arteriography, teach him how to cough forcefully and abruptly at appropriate intervals. Taking this step could save precious seconds in an emergency.

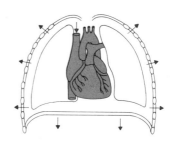

A deep breath lowers intrathoracic pressure, promoting venous return to the heart (above).

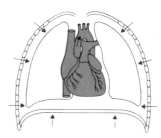

A deep cough raises intrathoracic pressure, increasing coronary perfusion (above).

Cardiac Arrest/Cardiac Trauma

Precordial thump

By inducing ventricular depolarization, the precordial thump may help convert ventricular dysrhythmias to sinus rhythm. Only two monitored situations warrant use of the precordial thump:
• the onset of ventricular tachycardia or ventricular fibrillation
• ventricular asystole that results from heart block in which rhythmic thumps produce a QRS complex and associated myocardial contraction (until a pacemaker can be inserted).

Important: Make sure you check your hospital's policy on this procedure. A precordial thump's no longer considered part of basic life support.

activity. For information on drugs commonly used during cardiac arrest, see pages 132 and 133.

In defibrillation, the treatment of choice for cardiac arrest induced by ventricular fibrillation, an electric current simultaneously depolarizes myocardial muscle fibers, causing synchronous myocardial contraction followed by repolarization. In theory, the sinoatrial (SA) node then produces a normal electrical impulse, which stimulates normal, coordinated cardiac rhythm.

Defibrillation should begin as soon as possible. However, the technique may fail if the myocardium grows extremely hypoxic, such as after the initial minutes of an arrest. If you don't know how long your patient's been in arrest, start BLS to reverse hypoxia—*then* defibrillate.

Defibrillation's also warranted for the cardiac arrest patient with ventricular tachycardia, if he's unconscious and lacks effective circulation; such a patient can't wait for health care workers to prepare for synchronized cardioversion. Although defibrillation generally won't help the patient with asystole, the doctor may use it when he can't distinguish fine defibrillation from true cardiac standstill.

Automatic implantable defibrillator (AID). Like many nurses, you may be seeing an increasing number of patients with a history of sudden death—ventricular fibrillation with a loss of consciousness. Studies show that these patients greatly risk further episodes of ventricular tachydysrhythmia. But the AID can help control ventricular fibrillation. This treatment generally supplements antiarrhythmic drugs, pacemakers, or both—or may be used after such therapies fail.

The doctor implants the AID (which has two defibrillator electrodes attached to its base generator) into the patient's abdominal cavity. He inserts the apical cardiac electrode through a left thoracotomy at the fifth intercostal space. Using fluoroscopy, he inserts the second electrode via the superior vena cava, positioning it near the right atrial junction.

Continued on page 136

Automatic implantable defibrillator (AID): Instant lifesaver

The AID, used to treat patients with recurrent life-threatening dysrhythmias, consists of a small pulse generator implanted in the patient's abdomen (see illustration at right). One of the unit's leads senses heart rate at the right ventricle; the second lead, which senses morphology, and thus rhythm, defibrillates at the right atrium; the third lead defibrillates at the apical pericardium. The AID can be programmed to suit each patient's needs, and it uses far less energy (25 joules on the first attempt) than does an external defibrillator (400 joules).

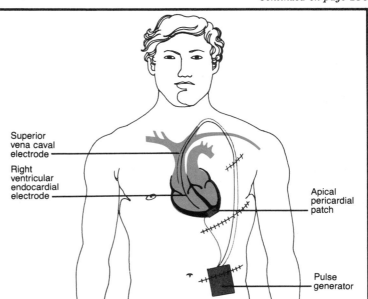

Superior vena caval electrode

Right ventricular endocardial electrode

Apical pericardial patch

Pulse generator

Cardiac Arrest/Cardiac Trauma

Near-death events (NDEs)

CPR's success has produced an unusual phenomenon—the remembrance of near-death events (NDEs) by patients surviving cardiac arrest.

Resuscitated patients have reported similar experiences and perceptions. Some say they felt relaxed, comfortable, and pain-free even though they believed they were dead. Others have described a mind-body separation, the mind observing resuscitation efforts from a corner of the room (known as autoscopic observation). Some patients report that their minds left the room (called transcendence). In some cases, patients have described events that only a resuscitation observer could have known.

With any patient who's just been resuscitated, offer support by gradually reorienting him to time, place, and person while you assess any changes in personality, memory, and thinking. When he's stable, discuss the resuscitation and encourage him to relate any NDEs he might have had. Like most patients who've had NDEs, he may not readily discuss the experience for fear of being thought "crazy", even if he feels a need to do so. Remember, a patient who's had an NDE perceives the event as real. Offer a supportive environment for discussion of his experience, and help him cope with his resuscitation memories. If necessary, refer him to counseling.

Cardiac arrest—*continued*

When the AID senses a ventricular tachydysrhythmia, it discharges a small shock (25 to 30 joules) to automatically defibrillate the heart, returning it to a sinus rhythm. If the initial discharge doesn't end the dysrhythmia, the AID can discharge up to four times, increasing the voltage each time. The unit usually lasts 3 years or up to 100 discharges.

Your main responsibility for a patient with an AID involves preoperative and postoperative care and patient teaching. Tell the patient that he'll have small incisions in the left side of his chest, right shoulder, and abdomen, and that he'll feel the unit discharging. (Some patients describe this as a sudden blow to the chest.) Warn the patient that during a true ventricular dysrhythmia, he'll experience sudden faintness or shortness of breath (or both), followed by the discharge and a return to a feeling of well-being. The episode usually lasts less than 30 seconds.

Newer AID models can also cardiovert such dysrhythmias as ventricular tachycardia and Torsades de Pointes. These models sense the absence of a true isoelectric line between QRS complexes as their discharging cue.

Evaluation

Your evaluation of the cardiac arrest patient's present condition will help determine his future care. Once he's been resuscitated and stabilized, begin a continuous and thorough assessment, including investigation of the cause of the arrest.

A complete evaluation should include psychological as well as physical assessment. Many resuscitated patients experience so-called near-death events (NDEs)—perceptions or recollections of events during the moment of clinical death. Keep this in mind *during* as well as after resuscitation, since the patient may be conscious of procedures and conversations around him. Help him confront these events later by giving emotional support and encouraging him to talk about them.

Also critique your role in the resuscitation effort. This step will leave you better prepared for the next cardiac arrest emergency.

Cardiac trauma

Cardiac trauma falls into two categories: blunt (nonpenetrating) and penetrating. Either type can damage the heart, its internal structures, the pericardium, and the great vessels (superior vena cava, inferior vena cava, and aorta).

Blunt trauma results from external force. The heart's position in the chest cavity—freely suspended by the great vessels—leaves it vulnerable to certain injury types. Blunt cardiac trauma most frequently results from sudden acceleration or deceleration (as in a steering wheel injury), which propels the heart into the sternum or vertebrae. A second cause, a forceful blow to the sternum (such as a fall from a great height), compresses the heart between the sternum and vertebrae. Another blunt injury type (for instance, from a blast) comes from a sudden, extreme rise in intrathoracic or intraabdominal pressure.

Cardiac Arrest/Cardiac Trauma

Blunt chest trauma most commonly leads to myocardial contusion. However, blunt trauma can also rupture the myocardium and great vessels (see *Guide to cardiac trauma* below).

Penetrating trauma results from a stab wound (from a knife or pick, for example) or from a missile (such as a bullet or shrapnel) that penetrates the heart and great vessels. Such trauma most often leads to a wound along the precordium, and usually involves the right ventricle—the most anterior cardiac chamber. This injury type

Continued on page 138

Guide to cardiac trauma

Injury: Myocardial contusion
Results in bruised myocardium; particularly affects the right ventricle because of this chamber's location

Possible causes:
Blunt chest trauma, particularly from a motor vehicle accident, which forces the chest against the steering wheel

Assessment:
• History of injury to anterior chest
• Ecchymosis on chest wall
• Shortness of breath
• Decreased blood pressure
• Chest pain
• Tachycardia
• Dysrhythmias—especially ventricular dysrhythmias or heart block
• EKG changes (up to 24 hours later) indicating apparent myocardial infarction (MI) or conduction disturbance
• Pericardial friction rub
• Signs and symptoms similar to those of MI or congestive heart failure

Diagnostic tests:
• Radionuclide studies
• Echocardiogram
• Serum CPK-MB

Interventions:
• Evaluate airway, breathing, and circulation (ABCs).
• Apply measures based on patient's signs and symptoms. (Treatments may include oxygen, analgesics, antiarrhythmics, and a pacemaker.)
• Prevent complications by watching for signs and symptoms of ruptured vessels or intracardiac structures, or cardiac tamponade. Avoid anticoagulants, which may precipitate myocardial bleeding.

Injury: Myocardial and great vessel rupture
Results in exsanguination, usually fatal

Possible causes:
Blunt or penetrating chest trauma. Blunt trauma may cause myocardial rupture from forceful compression of the heart against the vertebral column, or myocardial laceration by a bone fragment. Rupture of a great vessel may stem from sudden deceleration, as seen in myocardial contusion. In penetrating trauma, the penetrating object may cause injury.

Assessment:
• History of abrupt deceleration or compression injury, or penetrating chest wound
• Chest or back pain
• Signs and symptoms of shock
• Dyspnea
• Change in level of consciousness
• Increased blood pressure or pulse amplitude in arms
• Signs and symptoms of cardiac tamponade
• Pneumothorax or hemothorax
• Mediastinal widening

Diagnostic tests:
• Chest X-ray (which may show widened mediastinum)

Interventions:
• Evaluate ABCs.
• Administer oxygen.
• Apply MAST, as ordered.
• If injury stems from penetrating object, don't remove object.
• If object has been removed, apply direct pressure to control bleeding.
• The doctor will perform immediate surgery or emergency thoracotomy.

Injury: Cardiac tamponade
With slow pericardial fluid accumulation, patient may not have signs and symptoms. With rapid accumulation, cardiac output decreases from increased intrapericardial pressure, resulting in decreased diastolic filling.

Possible causes:
Blunt or penetrating chest trauma; complications of other disorders such as neoplastic disease, infection (which may lead to chronic tamponade); or invasive procedures such as cardiac catheterization or pacemaker insertion

Assessment:
• Beck's triad: decreased blood pressure, muffled heart sounds, increased central venous pressure (CVP)
• Distended neck veins
• Tachycardia
• Dyspnea
• Indications of decreased cardiac output
• Pulsus paradoxus (drop in systolic blood pressure greater than 10 to 15 mm Hg during normal inspiration)

Diagnostic tests:
Doctor usually makes diagnosis from patient's signs and symptoms and history of blunt or penetrating trauma

Interventions:
• Evaluate ABCs.
• Administer oxygen.
• Apply MAST as ordered.
• The doctor may perform pericardiocentesis.

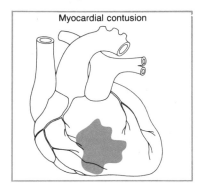
Myocardial contusion

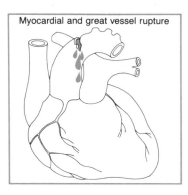
Myocardial and great vessel rupture

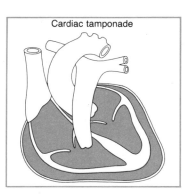
Cardiac tamponade

Cardiac Arrest/Cardiac Trauma

Danger: Pulsus paradoxus

Danger: Pulsus paradoxus

Always check a patient with a cardiac injury for pulsus paradoxus—a sign of cardiac tamponade. Pulsus paradoxus refers to a marked decrease in systolic blood pressure on inspiration. To assess pulsus paradoxus, inflate and then slowly deflate the blood pressure cuff until you hear the first systolic sound at expiration. Slowly continue to deflate the cuff until you hear sounds both on inspiration and expiration. The difference between the two readings is called the paradox. A difference greater than 10 mm Hg indicates pulsus paradoxus.

Cardiac trauma—*continued*

carries an extremely high death risk. Penetrating trauma that causes an open wound, exposing the heart and pericardium, can result in massive hemothorax. If the injury leaves a closed wound, in which the heart has been penetrated but the pericardium's not affected, cardiac tamponade can develop. (In some instances, tamponade exerts enough pressure on the wound to stifle hemorrhaging.)

Assessment

To assess cardiac trauma, first take a thorough patient history. In blunt trauma, obtain information about the impact; in penetrating trauma, obtain information about the direction of penetration and the type and length of the penetrating object.

Include the following steps in the physical examination:
• Fully inspect the patient's neck and anterior and posterior thorax
• Auscultate for changes in heart sounds and for murmur, S_3, or pulsus paradoxus
• Percuss the chest to assess heart size and thoracic fluid distribution
• Palpate the chest for tenderness and the neck for tracheal deviation (which may indicate a widened mediastinum).

Remember, as with all trauma patients, assess the patient's condition continuously, paying special attention to possible complications. (For specific signs and symptoms of trauma, see the chart on page 137.)

The doctor will diagnose cardiac trauma mainly from the patient's history and clinical condition.

Planning

When caring for a cardiac trauma patient, your priorities include ensuring adequate cardiac output and preventing cardiac tamponade.

Nursing diagnoses. Possible nursing diagnoses for a cardiac trauma patient include:
• cardiac output, alteration in (decreased); related to cardiac trauma
• gas exchange, impaired (potential for); related to chest injury

Sample nursing care plan—cardiac trauma

Nursing diagnosis	Expected outcomes
Cardiac output, alteration in (decreased); related to cardiac trauma	The patient will: • maintain adequate cardiac output • maintain adequate tissue perfusion.
Nursing interventions • Monitor vital signs, level of consciousness, and urine output for indications of decreased cardiac output. • Observe for adequate hemodynamic response after administration of blood, fluids, and pharmacologic products. • If patient's using MAST, assess his peripheral leg pulses. Inflate MAST until adequate cardiac output's obtained. Closely monitor patient's blood pressure and observe for respiratory impairment.	**Discharge planning** Depends on treatment outcome.

Cardiac Arrest/Cardiac Trauma

Reviewing pericardiocentesis

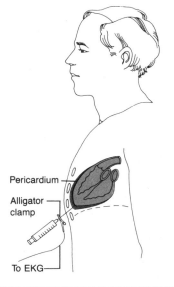

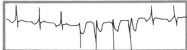

The doctor can perform pericardiocentesis at the patient's bedside by connecting an EKG's V, or chest, lead to a needle shank with an alligator clamp and ground wire. He'll probably insert the needle using a subxiphoid approach. Or he may insert it at the fifth intercostal space, lateral to the cardiac apex; to the left of the fifth or sixth intercostal space at the sternal margin; or to the right of the fourth intercostal space.

The doctor then slowly advances the needle, applying gentle intermittent suction on the syringe until he aspirates fluid. If premature ventricular contractions (PVCs) or elevated ST or PR segments appear on EKG (signs that the needle has contacted the myocardium), he'll withdraw the needle.

Note the amount and type of aspirated fluid. Pericardial blood has a lower hematocrit than venous blood, and won't clot when put in a test tube because the heart's motion defibrinates it.

In addition to myocardial injury, pericardiocentesis can lead to such complications as dysrhythmias; bacterial infection; subpericardial hematoma; and injury to the stomach, liver, or lungs.

• tissue perfusion, alteration in (decreased); related to decreased cardiac output.

The sample nursing care plan for a cardiac trauma patient on page 138 shows expected outcomes, nursing interventions, and discharge planning for one of the nursing diagnoses listed. Remember, though, to individualize each care plan to fit the patient's needs.

Intervention
The cardiac trauma patient usually requires immediate intervention. This may include emergency thoracotomy, pericardiocentesis, or surgical intervention, as well as measures that support cardiac output such as MAST and drugs.

Evaluation
Base your evaluation of the cardiac trauma patient on whether he responds to therapy.

Ask yourself the following questions based on the expected outcomes listed on the sample care plan on page 138, to determine your patient's response to treatment:
• Can the patient maintain adequate cardiac output?
• Does he show signs and symptoms of cardiac tamponade?
• Does he have adequate tissue perfusion?

The answers to these and other questions will help you evaluate the patient's condition and identify any complications. Keep in mind that these questions stem from the sample care plan. Your questions may vary.

Self Test

1. Which of the following actions should be your first priority during a cardiac arrest?
a. calling a code   **b.** beginning cardiopulmonary resuscitation   **c.** defibrillating the patient   **d.** determining the cause of the arrest

2. Metabolic acidosis occurring during a cardiac arrest may result from all of the following, except:
a. increased Purkinje fiber depolarization   **b.** heightened susceptibility to ventricular fibrillation   **c.** decreased ventricular contractile force   **d.** decreased cardiac responsiveness to catecholamines

3. When administering atropine to increase heart rate during a code, you'll normally give an initial dosage of:
a. 0.4 mg   **b.** 0.5 mg   **c.** 2.4 mg   **d.** 2.5 mg

4. Monitor the patient with a myocardial contusion for:
a. complete heart block   **b.** atrial fibrillation   **c.** sinus bradycardia **d.** premature atrial contractions

5. To assess a patient for pulsus paradoxus, check for:
a. a decrease in systolic blood pressure on inspiration   **b.** an increase in systolic blood pressure on inspiration   **c.** a decrease in systolic blood pressure on expiration   **d.** an increase in systolic blood pressure on expiration

Answers (page number shows where answer appears in text)

1. **b** (page 131)   2. **a** (page 134)   3. **b** (page 132)   4. **a** (page 137) 5. **a** (page 138)

Congenital Heart Defects: Structural Heart Abnormalities

Carol Langton and **Carolyn Vieweg** coauthored this chapter. A graduate of the Frankford Hospital School of Nursing, Philadelphia, Ms. Langton is head nurse in the cardiac intensive care unit at St. Christopher's Hospital for Children, Philadelphia. Ms. Vieweg is a clinical nurse specialist in cardiology and cardiothoracic surgery at St. Christopher's Hospital. She received her BSN from West Virginia University and her MSN from the University of Pittsburgh.

Congenital heart defects occur in about 8 to 10 of every 1,000 live births. Today, more affected infants survive, thanks to improved surgical procedures, new drugs, and other advances.

But we still have much to learn about these defects. For example, we rarely know for sure what causes them. Probably, they result from a complex interaction of genetic and environmental factors. Maternal rubella, alcoholism, malnutrition, and insulin-dependent diabetes may increase the risk. So may the ingestion of certain drugs by either parent. Other risk factors include a family history of such defects and concurrent chromosomal or other noncardiac anomalies.

The congenital heart defects we'll discuss in this chapter fall into

The heart's beginnings

The heart of a 3-week-old embryo consists of a six-part primitive cardiac tube. The truncus arteriosus develops into the aorta and pulmonary artery; the conus, into the crista supraventricularis. The bulbus cordis forms the right ventricle, while the primitive ventricle forms the left ventricle. The sinus venosus joins the primitive atrium to become the right and left atria.

At about the 4th week of gestation, the cardiac loop forms. The atria and ventricle then assume their final positions and the heart begins beating spontaneously. The atrial septum buds from the atrial roof and grows toward the endocardial cushions, between the mitral and tricuspid valves.

The atrial septum develops from two parts. The septum primum grows downward from the dorsal atrial wall, fuses with the endocardial cushion, and develops perforations that become the foramen ovale. The septum secundum arises from the superior atrial wall to the right of the septum primum.

At the same time, the ventricular septum grows upward to fuse with the endocardial cushion, completing the heart's four-chambered structure by the 6th to 8th week of gestation. The heart of the 7-week-old embryo resembles the adult's, but with two important exceptions: the ductus arteriosus and the foramen ovale, both essential for fetal circulation, remain patent.

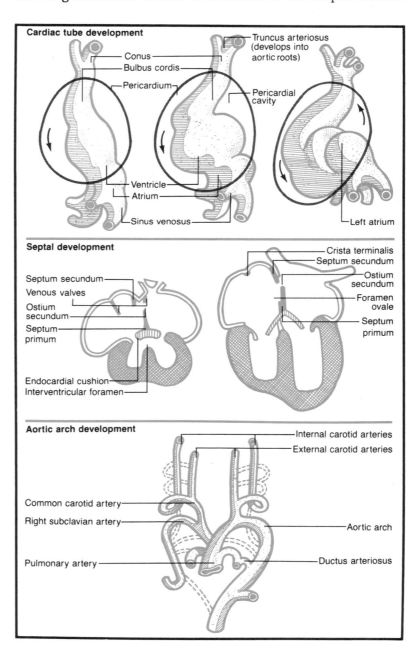

Cardiac tube development

Conus — Truncus arteriosus (develops into aortic roots)
Bulbus cordis
Pericardium
Pericardial cavity
Ventricle
Atrium
Sinus venosus
Left atrium

Septal development

Septum secundum — Crista terminalis
Septum secundum
Venous valves — Ostium secundum
Ostium secundum — Foramen ovale
Septum primum — Septum primum
Endocardial cushion
Interventricular foramen

Aortic arch development

Internal carotid arteries
External carotid arteries
Common carotid artery
Right subclavian artery
Aortic arch
Pulmonary artery
Ductus arteriosus

Congenital Heart Defects

two categories: acyanotic and cyanotic. *Acyanotic* defects include the following:
- aortic stenosis
- atrial septal defect (ASD)
- coarctation of the aorta
- endocardial cushion defect
- patent ductus arteriosus (PDA)
- pulmonary stenosis
- ventricular septal defect (VSD).

Acyanotic defects don't interfere with shunting of oxygenated blood from the heart's high-pressure left side to its low-pressure right side. As a result, the left ventricle continues ejecting oxygenated blood, preventing cyanosis.

Cyanotic defects include the following:
- hypoplastic left ventricle syndrome
- hypoplastic right ventricle syndrome
- persistent truncus arteriosus
- pulmonary atresia
- tetralogy of Fallot

Continued on page 142

Understanding fetal circulation

During fetal life, the placenta carries out oxygen and carbon dioxide exchange. Oxygenated blood flows from the placenta via the umbilical vein to the ductus venosus, into the inferior vena cava and on to the right atrium. Because the fetal heart's right side normally has higher pressure than its left side, this oxygenated blood shunts from the right atrium to the left atrium through the foramen ovale. It then flows into the left ventricle and through the aorta to the head and upper torso.

Unoxygenated blood returns to the right atrium through the superior vena cava, flows into the right ventricle, and exits through the pulmonary artery. Most of this blood shunts through the ductus arteriosus into the descending aorta, then travels to the placenta via the umbilical artery. However, some blood also flows to and from the lungs.

At birth, umbilical cord clamping and lung expansion cause profound circulatory changes. Lung expansion increases pulmonary blood flow and reduces pulmonary vascular resistance, which elevates left atrial pressure and decreases right ventricular pressure. As a result, the ductus venosus, foramen ovale, and ductus arteriosus close, and extrauterine circulation begins. The lungs then take over oxygen and carbon dioxide exchange.

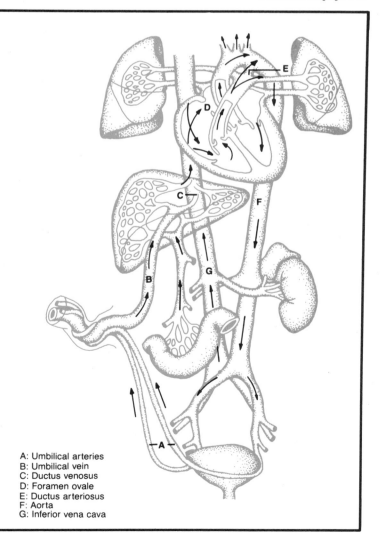

A: Umbilical arteries
B: Umbilical vein
C: Ductus venosus
D: Foramen ovale
E: Ductus arteriosus
F: Aorta
G: Inferior vena cava

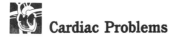

Congenital Heart Defects

Developmental stages and age-related fears

When planning nursing care for the child with a congenital heart defect, always consider his age and developmental level. For example, a preschooler fears body injury and pain, so be sure to provide support and reassurance when giving injections or performing other invasive procedures. The table below shows major fears associated with various developmental stages.

Infants
Developmental stage
Trust versus mistrust
Major fear
Separation

Toddlers
Developmental stage
Autonomy versus shame and doubt
Major fears
Separation
Loss of control
1. Physical limitation
2. Loss of rituals

Preschoolers
Developmental stage
Initiative versus guilt
Major fears
Separation
Loss of control
Body injury and pain—fear of intrusive procedures and mutilation

School-aged children
Developmental stage
Industry versus inferiority
Major fears
Separation
1. Parents
2. Peers
Loss of control
Body injury and pain

Modified from Erikson, E.: *Childhood and Society.* New York: W.W. Norton & Co., 1963

Continued
- total anomalous pulmonary venous return
- complete transposition of the great vessels (TGV)
- tricuspid atresia.

How does cyanosis develop? Abnormally high pressure in the heart's right side allows right-to-left shunting of unoxygenated blood. This blood then mixes with oxygenated blood, resulting in arterial blood oxygen desaturation. Inadequate pulmonary blood flow may also contribute to cyanosis. Chronic arterial oxygen desaturation leads to polycythemia, which increases the risk of thrombus formation and cerebrovascular accident. (Take special precautions with I.V. lines when caring for a child with a cyanotic heart defect; air or a dislodged clot entering the systemic circulation could cause an arterial embolus.)

Assessment

Your assessment of the patient with a congenital heart defect includes the normal cardiac assessment—and much more. Because the patient's age can range from newborn to adult, you'll have to recognize his age-related physical and psychological needs and developmental level. And, as always, evaluate the family's needs. Do family members fully accept the patient's diagnosis? Do they understand the heart defect? How do they expect treatment to help? Recognize that the patient's diagnosis may cause a family crisis, especially if the patient's an infant or a young child. (For assessment information about specific defects, see pages 144 to 156.)

Planning

Formulate your care plan with these two goals in mind: maintaining adequate oxygenation and cardiac output and preventing compli-

---

Sample nursing care plan—congenital heart defect

Nursing diagnosis	Expected outcomes
Knowledge deficit related to the diagnosis of congenital heart defect.	• The patient (if appropriate) and his family will show knowledge of the defect, including its medical and surgical management. • The family will participate in care planning and implementation.

Nursing interventions	Discharge planning
• Orient the patient and his family to the hospital. • Consult with the doctor about his plan for the patient. • Reinforce the doctor's plan in words that the patient and his family can understand. • Explain necessary procedures and encourage the patient and his family to ask questions. • Assess the patient's and family's preparation for surgery and plan a teaching approach. • Encourage the patient and his family to tell you what they know about the defect. • Assess the patient's and family's willingness to learn. • Establish a trusting relationship with the patient. • Encourage the family to participate in the patient's care. • Provide emotional support. • Document the patient's and family's strengths and weaknesses.	• Reinforce the treatment plan. • Teach the patient and his family about medications and other therapeutic measures. • Emphasize the need for follow-up care and arrange for such care if appropriate. • Refer the family to community health agencies and support groups, if appropriate.

Congenital Heart Defects

cations. Once these goals have been met, direct your efforts toward educating the patient (if he's old enough to understand) and his family about the heart defect and providing emotional support. Carefully consider the patient's age when planning care.

Nursing diagnoses. The nursing diagnoses that may make up your care plan include the following:
• knowledge deficit related to diagnosis of congenital heart defect
• cardiac output, alteration in (decreased); related to dysrhythmia, hypovolemia, decreased myocardial function
• tissue perfusion, alteration in (decreased); related to decreased cardiac output
• fluid volume, alteration in (excess); related to the heart's decreased pumping ability
• gas exchange, impaired; related to excess fluid volume
• anxiety related to hospitalization, disease process
• family dynamics, alteration in; related to disease
• coping, ineffective family; related to disease
• activity intolerance related to decreased cardiac output, dyspnea, pain
• nutrition, alteration in: less than body requirements (potential for); related to surgery, respiratory impairment.

The sample nursing care plan for a congenital heart defect patient (on page 142) shows expected outcomes, nursing interventions, and discharge planning based on one nursing diagnosis. Remember, though, to tailor each care plan to the needs of the patient and his family.

Intervention
Nearly 25% of congenital heart defects produce symptoms in the first year of life, making early intervention essential. Medical management typically involves drugs that help control complications, such as congestive heart failure. Surgical intervention may be palliative or corrective. In either case, you'll be expected to prepare the patient physically and emotionally and to help prevent postoperative complications. (See pages 145 to 156 to review interventions for specific defects; see the chart on pages 154 and 155 to review possible complications of corrective surgery.)

New advances. Recent interventions include the intraaortic balloon pump (IABP) and heart transplantation. With IABP, the doctor inserts the inflatable balloon percutaneously through the external iliac artery, then advances it into the aorta just below the level of the left subclavian artery. The balloon provides intermittent counterpulsation during diastole, which improves coronary artery blood flow and reduces peripheral vascular resistance. Although used extensively in adults, this device has recently been adapted for children through modifications in the balloon's size and in the pumping rate. It's now commonly used as a temporary measure in children with severe cardiac dysfunction before and immediately after cardiac surgery. The IABP markedly improves the child's cardiac index and survival odds. However, stay alert for such complications as bleeding, thromboemboli, leg ischemia, and decreased mesenteric or renal artery perfusion. (See Chapter 5 for more information about the IABP).

Continued on page 144

Congenital Heart Defects

Continued

Currently reserved for end-stage heart disease, heart transplantation involves removal of the child's diseased heart, except for the posterior right and left atrial walls and their venous connections. After anastomosing the donor's heart to the child's remaining atrial tissue, the surgical team joins the donor's pulmonary artery and aorta with the stumps of the patient's same vessels. The patient's immune system normally recognizes the transplanted heart as a foreign substance and fights to reject it. On the average, an acute rejection episode occurs twice in the month after transplantation. Stay alert for chest pain, lethargy, fever, and personality changes, which may signal an acute rejection episode.

The immunosuppressant cyclosporine (Sandimmune) has dramatically improved survival rates after heart transplantation. Steroids and periodic endomyocardial biopsy to detect cellular rejection also contribute to success. The 1-year survival rate after heart transplantation approaches 70%; the 5-year survival rate nears 50%. (See Chapter 5 for more information about heart transplantation.)

Evaluation

Evaluate the patient with a congenital heart defect according to the expected outcomes in your care plan. To determine if his condition's improved, ask yourself the following questions:
• Do the patient (if appropriate) and his family understand the congenital heart defect?
• Do they understand the treatment plan?
• If surgery's scheduled, have they received adequate preoperative and postoperative teaching?
• Do they participate in care planning and implementation?

The answers to these and other questions will help you evaluate your patient's condition and the effectiveness of his care. Keep in mind that these questions stem from the care plan on page 142. Your questions may differ.

Acyanotic heart defects

We'll review the following acyanotic defects: ventricular septal defect, patent ductus arteriosus, atrial septal defect, endocardial cushion defect, and coarctation of the aorta. (For information about aortic and pulmonary stenosis, see Chapter 7.)

Ventricular septal defect

In this disorder, the most common congenital heart defect, an abnormal communication or opening in the ventricular septum allows blood to shunt from the left to right ventricle. It may be associated with other defects, such as tetralogy of Fallot, transposition of the great vessels, and coarctation of the aorta.

A VSD occurs when membranous and/or muscular tissues don't fuse properly with the endocardial cushions and bulbus cordis during the 4th to 8th weeks of gestation. Usually, the defect occurs in the membranous or muscular portion of the ventricular septum. The opening can range from pinpoint size to the entire absence of the septum, although large defects occur relatively infrequently. Approximately 50% close spontaneously by age 2.

Initially, blood shunts from the left to right ventricle, resulting in

Complete endocardial cushion defect

This condition arises when the common channel between the atria and ventricles fails to partition during embryonic development. This results in anomalies of the atrial and ventricular septa and the tricuspid and mitral valves. Also known as complete atrioventricular canal defect, this defect's commonly associated with trisomy 21.

Typically, neonates with complete endocardial cushion defect develop severe congestive heart failure and cyanosis. Most require corrective surgery in the first few years of life to prevent irreversible pulmonary hypertension. Such surgery involves prosthetic reconstruction of an atrial and ventricular septum and suturing of the mitral and tricuspid valves to the patch.

Congenital Heart Defects

Ventricular septal defect

In this disorder, an abnormal opening in the membranous (A) or muscular (B) portion of the ventricular septum allows oxygenated blood to shunt from the left to right ventricle (see illustration below).

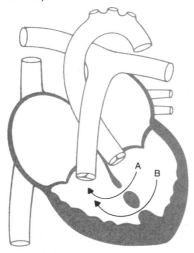

A: Membranous VSD
B: Muscular VSD

A role for drugs

Drugs that dilate or close the ductus arteriosus can help treat congenital heart defects. Prostaglandin E₁ (alprostadil, or Prostin VR) dilates the ductus, keeping it patent. This can improve pulmonary blood flow and oxygenation in cyanotic defects and systemic blood flow in certain acyanotic defects.

By inhibiting prostaglandin synthesis, indomethacin (Indocin) can close a patent ductus arteriosus. I.V. Indocin has been approved for certain premature infants who don't respond to other medical measures.

increased pulmonary blood flow. With a large defect, dramatic shunting may cause pulmonary vessel hypertrophy and increased pulmonary vascular resistance. This, in turn, elevates pulmonary and right ventricular pressure. When right ventricular pressure equals or exceeds left ventricular pressure, unoxygenated blood shunts from the right to left ventricle—a condition known as Eisenmenger's syndrome.

Assessment. Most infants don't have symptoms at birth because the right ventricle's pressure equals the left's, preventing shunting through the defect. When shunting begins, you'll auscultate a fixed systolic murmur at the lower left sternal border. If the defect's small, this murmur may go undetected until the infant becomes a preschooler. A child with a large VSD may develop congestive heart failure, feeding difficulties, frequent upper respiratory infections, shortness of breath, tachypnea, and diaphoresis at an earlier age. A moderate VSD causes poor weight gain and fatigue but no congestive heart failure findings.

A chest X-ray or EKG may reveal mild left ventricular hypertrophy, while an echocardiogram shows left atrial enlargement, which results from the large volume of pulmonary venous blood return. Cardiac catheterization determines the defect's size and location.

Intervention. The doctor will probably follow an asymptomatic child with a small to moderate VSD on an outpatient basis to give the defect time to close spontaneously. If the VSD remains patent, the child will undergo elective surgery at age 4 or 5—unless he becomes symptomatic, making earlier surgery necessary. A child with a large VSD usually requires treatment after the age of 1 month. Digitalis and diuretics help control signs and symptoms of congestive heart failure. If these drugs don't work and the infant weighs less than 4.4 lb (2 kg), the doctor may perform palliative surgery known as *pulmonary artery banding*. Using a thoracotomy, he wraps a Dacron strip around the main pulmonary artery to decrease pulmonary blood flow and prevent irreversible pulmonary vascular disease. Possible complications include congestive heart failure and low cardiac output syndrome.

The doctor probably won't perform surgical repair through a median sternotomy with cardiopulmonary bypass until the child reaches late preschool age. Then, sutures can effectively close a small defect; a Dacron patch repairs a larger one. Typically, the asymptomatic child has a better prognosis than the child with preoperative congestive heart failure and pulmonary hypertension.

Patent ductus arteriosus

The second most common congenital heart defect, PDA may be associated with rubella syndrome or other anomalies.

The ductus arteriosus—the fetal blood vessel connecting the aorta and pulmonary artery—allows blood to bypass nonfunctioning fetal lungs. When the infant begins breathing at birth, pulmonary vascular resistance decreases, causing dilation of the pulmonary vasculature. This, in turn, increases oxygen's partial pressure, causing ductus arteriosus constriction in the first 72 hours after birth. Normally, the ductus closes completely within 12 weeks. However, hypoxia and ductal scarring associated with rubella may prevent

Continued on page 146

Congenital Heart Defects

Patent ductus arteriosus

Normally, the ductus arteriosus—a fetal blood vessel connecting the aorta with the pulmonary artery—closes shortly after birth. In patent ductus arteriosus, this vessel remains open, allowing blood to shunt from the aorta to the pulmonary artery (as shown below).

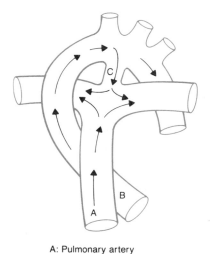

A: Pulmonary artery
B: Aorta
C: Patent ductus arteriosus

Acyanotic heart defects—*continued*

closure. Because aortic pressure exceeds pulmonary arterial pressure after birth, oxygenated blood shunts through the PDA from the aorta to the pulmonary artery and lungs. Thus, the PDA may save the life of an infant with associated cyanotic heart defects and decreased pulmonary blood flow.

Assessment. The shunt's size determines which signs and symptoms appear. The child with a small shunt may lack symptoms except for a classic "machinery" murmur during systole and diastole. You may also palpate a thrill over the suprasternal notch. In a patient with a larger shunt, check for bounding peripheral pulses and widened pulse pressure. He may also have signs and symptoms of congestive heart failure or respiratory distress. As he matures, he'll likely have recurrent respiratory infections and tire easily.

A chest X-ray may show cardiomegaly and increased pulmonary vascular markings. Although an EKG may not detect a small shunt, it may reveal left ventricular hypertrophy in a larger one. Echocardiography and cardiac catheterization help confirm the diagnosis.

Intervention. The doctor may delay surgical repair (generally the treatment of choice) in the critically ill neonate who's a poor surgical risk. Usually, he'll order fluid restrictions and diuretics to minimize the effects of congestive heart failure.

Later, during closed-heart surgery through a left thoracotomy, he'll ligate or divide the ductus. (An adult with a fragile, calcified ductus may require cardiopulmonary bypass.)

Indomethacin, a prostaglandin synthetase inhibitor, can also help close the ductus. However, this anti-inflammatory drug probably won't be given if the child has an infection. The drug may depress the bone marrow and decrease renal blood flow.

Atrial septal defect

The most common congenital heart defect diagnosed in adults, this abnormal opening in the atrial septum permits blood to shunt from the left to right atrium.

The atrial septum has two components: the muscular embryogenic septum secundum, which has a round posteroinferior opening called the foramen ovale; and the fibrous septum primum, with a round anterosuperior opening. The two overlap, acting as a one-way valve. Before birth, blood flows from the right to left atrium through the foramen ovale. After birth, left heart pressure increases, causing the overlapping sections to close and fuse together. If they fail to fuse, one of three major defects may occur:
• ostium secundum defect. The most common ASD, this occurs near the foramen ovale.
• sinus venosus defect. Usually associated with partial anomalous pulmonary venous return, this defect arises in the upper atrial septum next to the superior vena cava.
• ostium primum defect. This disorder, also known as incomplete endocardial cushion defect, takes place in the lower atrial septum, usually in association with a VSD or mitral insufficiency. Because left atrial pressure exceeds right atrial pressure, oxygenated blood shunts from the left to right atrium through the defect. This in-

Congenital Heart Defects

Atrial septal defects

An atrial septal defect (ASD)—an abnormal opening between the atria—allows shunting of blood from the left to right atrium. This defect can be classified as sinus venosus ASD, located in the upper atrial septum (A); ostium secundum ASD, located in the foramen ovale (B); or ostium primum ASD, located in the lower atrial septum (C).

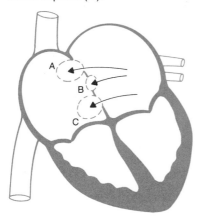

A: Sinus venosus ASD
B: Ostium secundum ASD
C: Ostium primum ASD

creases blood flow to the right heart and pulmonary arteries, causing right atrial and ventricular enlargement. Pulmonary hypertension rarely affects children unless other anomalies accompany the ASD, although it may affect adults with untreated ASD.

Assessment. Most patients lack symptoms until they reach the late teens or early adulthood. Then, expect complaints of fatigue and dyspnea on exertion. (However, you may auscultate a systolic murmur and a fixed split during a well-baby examination.) A chest X-ray may show cardiomegaly; EKG findings include right-axis deviation, peaked P waves, and right bundle branch block. Cardiac catheterization confirms the diagnosis.

Intervention. Surgical repair, the treatment of choice, typically brings excellent results. After placing the child on cardiopulmonary bypass, the doctor closes the ASD with sutures or a patch graft (for larger defects or for sinus venosus defect).

Coarctation of the aorta

This defect involves aortic narrowing or constriction. It may be associated with other cardiac defects, such as a VSD, an ASD, or a bicuspid aortic valve.

The disorder results from faulty development of the aortic arch in the 5th to 8th weeks of gestation. Although it may occur anywhere on the aortic arch, it usually develops just proximal to the ductus arteriosus (preductal coarctation). This encourages the ductus to remain open. If the defect occurs distal to the ductus arteriosus (postductal coarctation), the ductus narrows or closes.

In preductal coarctation, fetal circulation continues after birth, with blood from the right ventricle flowing through the ductus arteriosus into the descending aorta to the lower body. Blood from the left ventricle travels through the ascending aorta to the head and upper torso. This circulatory pattern strains the right heart, eventually enlarging the right ventricle, pulmonary artery, and descending aorta.

In postductal coarctation, collateral circulation develops in the proximal arteries during fetal life to bypass the coarcted segment, thereby supplying blood to the lower body. High pressure within the aorta proximal to the coarctation enlarges the left atrium and ventricle.

Assessment. Most infants with preductal coarctation have serious associated cardiac defects, such as hypoplastic left ventricle syndrome and VSD. So expect signs and symptoms of congestive heart failure during the first month of life. Check for systolic hypertension in the arms and systolic hypotension in the legs; the extremities will have similar diastolic pressures. On palpation, expect weak or absent femoral pulses, delayed after the radial pulse. You'll also note cyanosis in the legs, which receive unoxygenated blood from the right ventricle via the ductus arteriosus. Auscultate for a systolic ejection murmur at the left sternal border.

A chest X-ray may reveal cardiomegaly and increased pulmonary vascular markings. The EKG may identify right ventricular hypertrophy. Cardiac catheterization shows abnormal pressure gradients

Continued on page 148

Congenital Heart Defects

How coarctation diverts aortic blood flow

In coarctation of the aorta, narrowing or constriction occurs near the site where the aorta and ductus arteriosus join. If narrowing occurs proximal to this site (preductal coarctation), the ductus arteriosus remains open (top illustration). If narrowing occurs distal to this site (postductal coarctation), the ductus arteriosus closes, creating the *ligamentum arteriosum*, a fetal remnant (bottom illustration). Collateral circulation then develops to compensate for diminished blood flow beyond the coarctation.

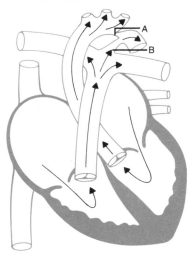

Coarctation of the aorta (preductal)

A: Preductal coarctation
B: Patent ductus arteriosus

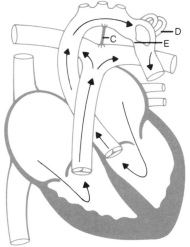

Coarctation of the aorta (postductal)

C: Ligamentum arteriosum
D: Collateral circulation
E: Postductal coarctation

Acyanotic heart defects—*continued*

within the heart and determines the size of the coarctation and of other associated defects.

In rare cases, you'll note signs and symptoms of congestive heart failure in postductal coarctation. Usually, this defect becomes apparent during routine physical examination of the school-age child or adolescent. Typically, the child appears pink instead of cyanotic. Check for blood pressure that's higher in the arms than in the legs. Also palpate for full peripheral arm pulses and weak or absent leg pulses. Ask about dyspnea and exercise intolerance. Does the child have leg claudication when he exercises? This reflects limited blood flow associated with collateral circulation. Some children also complain of headaches, nosebleeds, and cool feet. Auscultate for a continuous systolic murmur over the back, near the left thoracic vertebrae border, associated with collateral circulation. However, expect normal heart sounds.

A chest X-ray reveals an enlarged left atrium and ventricle and a dilated ascending aorta. In a child older than age 8, the X-ray may also show rib notching associated with collateral circulation. The EKG may be normal or may show left ventricular hypertrophy.

Intervention. The infant with congestive heart failure routinely receives digitalis and diuretics, perhaps combined with antihypertensive therapy. If these drugs prove ineffective, the doctor may perform surgery. Otherwise, he'll delay surgery until the child reaches at least age 3; by then, the aorta has grown to nearly adult size and hypertension can still be reversed.

The doctor will use one of the corrective surgical procedures described below, depending on the child's age and overall health and the defect's extent. Usually, each procedure takes place through a left thoracotomy incision without cardiopulmonary bypass. However, a child who's less than age 1 or who has poor collateral circulation may require cardiopulmonary bypass with hypothermia. Surgical procedures include:
- *end-to-end anastomosis* (recommended for children older than age 3). After clamping the aorta, the doctor resects the narrowed segment and performs an end-to-end anastomosis.
- *patch aortoplasty* (recommended for children older than age 3). After clamping the aorta, the doctor incises the vessel from the left subclavian artery, excises the coarcted segment, and sews a large Dacron patch over the aorta. The patch eliminates the risk of circular anastomosis constriction, which may develop with end-to-end anastomosis.
- *subclavian flap aortoplasty.* After clamping the aorta, the doctor ligates the left distal segment of the subclavian artery and incises it laterally. He then incises the aorta's coarcted segment, flaps the left distal segment of the subclavian artery down to the aorta, and sutures it in place. This procedure decreases the time required for cross-clamping the aorta and allows the flapped tissue to grow with the child.

Cyanotic heart defects

We'll discuss the following cyanotic defects: tetralogy of Fallot, complete transposition of the great vessels, tricuspid atresia, hy-

Congenital Heart Defects

Tetralogy of Fallot: Four defects in one

Tetralogy of Fallot combines four specific defects, as shown below: ventricular septal defect (A), overriding of the aorta (B), pulmonary stenosis (C), and right ventricular hypertrophy (D).

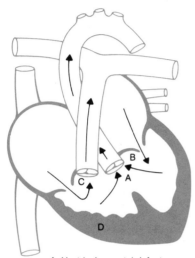

A: Ventricular septal defect
B: Aorta overriding the VSD
C: Pulmonary artery stenosis
D: Right ventricular hypertrophy

poplastic left ventricle syndrome, persistent truncus arteriosus, and total anomalous pulmonary venous return.

Tetralogy of Fallot

The most common cyanotic heart defect, tetralogy of Fallot combines four specific defects: VSD, pulmonary stenosis, overriding of the aorta, and right ventricular hypertrophy. Presumably, pulmonary stenosis and overriding of the aorta result from faulty development of the subpulmonary conus. Right ventricular hypertrophy develops as pulmonary stenosis forces the right ventricle to work harder. VSD results from conal septum misalignment.

The degree of pulmonary stenosis determines the hemodynamic changes this defect causes. Mild pulmonary stenosis slightly increases right ventricular pressure, resulting in a left-to-right shunt. This causes noncyanotic, or "pink", tetralogy. More severe pulmonary stenosis markedly increases right ventricular pressure, resulting in a right-to-left shunt. Pulmonary stenosis may be so severe that the child's life depends on a PDA to provide pulmonary blood flow.

Assessment. Cyanosis, a hallmark of tetralogy of Fallot, usually develops within several months of birth. However, it may occur later in an infant with a PDA or initially mild pulmonary stenosis. Cyanosis becomes especially marked during *tet*, or hypoxic, spells. These spells, which presumably result from spasm of the right ventricular outflow tract, may arise after activities that increase oxygen demand and pulmonary vascular resistance, such as bowel movements, feeding, and agitation. Initially, spells remain brief but may later become prolonged, resulting in unconsciousness, seizures, or death.

During your assessment, ask about decreased exercise tolerance—a common indication. Dyspnea typically occurs during feeding or crying. The child may squat when he feels short of breath during play or mild exercise; apparently, this position reduces right-to-left shunting. Also check for polycythemia and clubbed fingers—signs of chronic hypoxemia. The child may be small and poorly developed for his age. Auscultate for a systolic ejection murmur along the left sternal border. Also check for a continuous murmur across the child's back—a result of collateral circulation to the lungs.

An EKG will show right ventricular hypertrophy, right axis deviation, and occasionally peaked P waves. The chest X-ray reveals a normal size heart with decreased pulmonary blood flow. Elevation of the heart's apex will make the organ appear boot-shaped. Cardiac catheterization reveals normal right atrial pressure and equal right and left ventricular pressures; it can also establish the degree of pulmonary stenosis.

Intervention. Medical management aims to prevent or treat tet spells through the use of morphine sulfate (0.1 mg/kg), Inderal (0.5 to 2 mg/kg), and oxygen therapy. Placing the child in a knees-to-chest or squatting position may also improve oxygenation. If metabolic acidosis results from hypoxia, the doctor will also order sodium bicarbonate. Encourage adequate fluid intake to prevent hemoconcentration associated with polycythemia. Warn the parents that the patient should be given prophylactic antibiotics even for minor sur-

Continued on page 150

Congenital Heart Defects

Persistent truncus arteriosus

Normally, the embryonic truncus arteriosus forks into the aorta and the pulmonary artery. When this division doesn't occur—a defect known as persistent truncus arteriosus—a single vessel supplies both pulmonary and systemic blood flow.

Hemodynamic changes stemming from truncus arteriosus depend on the patient's pulmonary arterial status. Normal size arteries allow excessive pulmonary blood flow, resulting in cardiac or pulmonary failure and slight cyanosis. Stenotic arteries precipitate more dramatic cyanosis but fewer signs and symptoms of heart failure.

Besides indications of congestive heart failure, note any growth retardation when examining the child. Auscultate for a systolic murmur at the left sternal border and for a continuous murmur over both lung fields. You may also hear a single second heart sound and a constant ejection sound. A diastolic murmur, a grim prognostic sign, indicates truncal valve insufficiency.

A chest X-ray will reveal cardiomegaly and increased pulmonary vascular markings. Echocardiography may confirm the diagnosis. Cardiac catheterization visualizes the defect and measures pulmonary arterial resistance.

Medical management aims to control congestive heart failure. Surgery involves pulmonary artery banding or ventricular septal defect closure with insertion of a valved conduit between the right ventricle and pulmonary artery.

Cyanotic heart defects—*continued*

gical procedures to reduce the risk of bacterial endocarditis.

Doctors disagree about the best surgical approach for tetralogy of Fallot. Some recommend immediate corrective surgery, regardless of the child's age. Others prefer palliative surgery first, in the symptomatic child who's too small for corrective surgery. Palliative surgery establishes a systemic pulmonary artery shunt to reduce hypoxia.

The most frequently used surgery, the Blalock-Taussig shunt, involves anastomosis of the subclavian artery to the pulmonary artery, with collateral circulation maintaining blood flow to the arm. Occasionally, the procedure's modified by connecting the subclavian and pulmonary arteries with a polytetrafluoroethylene graft. This shunt increases pulmonary blood flow but not excessively, because the subclavian artery's size restricts blood flow somewhat. However, the child may outgrow the shunt, making a second operation necessary.

In rare cases, the doctor may perform the Potts' shunt—anastomosis of the descending aorta to the pulmonary artery. This procedure gives poor control of pulmonary blood flow and, during a total repair, the shunt proves hard to close. Another rarely used procedure, the Waterston shunt, involves anastomosis of the ascending aorta to the pulmonary artery. This technique also gives poor control of pulmonary blood flow and may cause pulmonary artery constriction.

Corrective surgery requires a median sternotomy incision. After removing any palliative shunts, the doctor places the child on cardiopulmonary bypass. He then resects the pulmonary infundibular muscle and performs a pulmonary valvotomy. If the pulmonary outflow tract's small, he may place a Dacron or pericardial patch across it or establish a conduit between the right ventricle and pulmonary artery. He'll close the VSD with a Dacron patch.

Less than 10% of children with uncorrected tetralogy of Fallot survive to age 21. Those undergoing corrective surgery have an excellent prognosis, except for a slightly increased incidence of sudden death years later. This risk increases in the patient with right ventricular hypertension or right bundle branch block. Restricted pulmonary blood flow results in more postoperative deaths than any other single cause.

Complete transposition of the great vessels

Also known as transposition of the great arteries (TGA), this defect constitutes the second most common cyanotic heart defect.

In TGV, the aorta leaves the right ventricle and the pulmonary artery leaves the left ventricle, producing two independent blood circuits. (In dextrotransposition, or D-transposition, the most common TGV form, the aorta sits in front and to the right of the pulmonary artery.) Unoxygenated blood flows through the right atrium and ventricle, then out the transposed aorta to the systemic circulation. Oxygenated blood flows from the lungs through the left atrium and ventricle, then out the transposed pulmonary artery

Congenital Heart Defects

When the great arteries change places

In transposition of the great vessels (TGV), the aorta arises from the right ventricle and the pulmonary artery from the left ventricle, creating two independent circulatory systems (pulmonary and systemic). However, slight blood mixing occurs at the patent foramen ovale and the patent ductus arteriosus, as shown below.

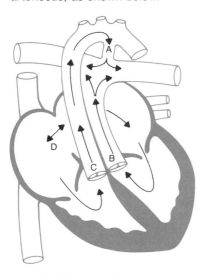

A: Patent ductus arteriosus
B: Pulmonary artery
C: Aorta
D: Patent foramen ovale

back to the lungs. TGV may quickly cause death unless the infant has associated cardiac defects that allow pulmonary and systemic blood to mix. About 50% of infants with TGV initially have a patent ductus arteriosus and/or a patent foramen ovale. Another 30% have a VSD, which allows even greater blood mixing.

TGV results from faulty embryonic development of the truncus arteriosus, which normally divides to form the aorta and pulmonary artery during the 3rd and 4th weeks of gestation. The aorta and pulmonary artery normally migrate to their respective places in the ventricle.

Usually, the infant with TGV has cyanosis at birth, the severity of the disorder depending on the degree of pulmonary and systemic blood mixing. A patent foramen ovale allows mixing between the atria; a PDA allows mixing between the pulmonary artery and aorta. However, when the ductus arteriosus constricts and closes 2 to 3 days after birth, the infant may become profoundly cyanotic and acidotic. A VSD allows blood mixing between the ventricles. Eventually, though, chronic cyanosis may lead to polycythemia, tissue hypoxia, and metabolic acidosis, which demand immediate intervention.

Assessment. Besides characteristic cyanosis, the infant may show signs and symptoms of congestive heart failure if he has a large associated VSD. Also assess for other common indications, including tachypnea, tet spells, failure to feed, dyspnea, and hepatomegaly. In a few cases, you may auscultate a soft murmur at the midsternal border.

An EKG may show right ventricular hypertrophy, right axis deviation, or right atrial enlargement. Although initially normal, a chest X-ray eventually reveals increased pulmonary vascular markings. Right atrial and ventricular enlargement make the heart look like an egg on its side. Echocardiography confirms the diagnosis by showing reversal of the aorta and pulmonary artery. Cardiac catheterization also confirms the abnormal positions and may reveal a PDA, VSD, or patent foramen ovale.

Intervention. Initially, the infant receives digitalis and diuretics to combat congestive heart failure. The doctor may give I.V. prostaglandin E_1 (alprostadil, or Prostin VR) to a hypoxic infant to keep the ductus arteriosus patent and improve systemic blood flow. Oxygen therapy and other measures help minimize tet spells (see the "Tetralogy of Fallot" section above). Supplemental iron given before major surgery helps prevent anemia.

Palliative procedures to reduce hypoxia, cyanosis, and congestive heart failure in TGV include the Rashkind balloon atrioseptostomy, pulmonary artery banding, and/or Blalock-Hanlon atrial septectomy.

• *Rashkind balloon atrioseptostomy.* Commonly performed during diagnostic cardiac catheterization on the infant's first day of life, this procedure involves passage of a 5 or 6 French double-lumen catheter through the right atrium into the left. The balloon catheter, gradually inflated and rapidly pulled across the foramen ovale two to five times, creates a moderate opening between the atria. Initially,

Continued on page 152

Congenital Heart Defects

Total anomalous pulmonary venous return

In this condition, a defect between the pulmonary veins and the systemic veins or right atrium causes abnormal venous drainage. Systemic and pulmonary venous blood mix in the right atrium, then flow into the left atrium, resulting in cyanosis. Cyanosis may appear within the first few days of life or later.

Besides cyanosis, assess for congestive heart failure and other common signs, such as pror weight gain and chronic tachypnea. Auscultate for a systolic murmur at the left sternal border and for prominent third and fourth heart sounds.

The chest X-ray will show the characteristic "snowman" configuration of the heart, with pulmonary venous drainage into the left innominate vein. Echocardiography may also outline the anomalous drainage route. Cardiac catheterization confirms the diagnosis and establishes the degree of pulmonary venous obstruction.

The doctor will use therapies that minimize the effects of congestive heart failure. Before undertaking surgery, he may perform balloon atrioseptostomy to increase blood mixing. Subsequent corrective surgery involves three steps: ligation of the anomalous venous defect, anastomosis of the pulmonary veins to the left atrium, and closure of the intraatrial defect.

Cyanotic heart defects—*continued*

this procedure dramatically improves oxygen saturation. But saturation eventually decreases and stabilizes at 40% to 50%. Prostaglandin therapy can then be gradually reduced, and corrective surgery done a few months later. In about 10% of infants, this procedure causes complications, such as dysrhythmia, tamponade, and heart perforation.

- *Pulmonary artery banding.* See page 145.

- *Blalock-Hanlon atrial septectomy.* This low-risk procedure establishes a large interatrial septal defect through excision of the interatrial septum's posterior portion. This reduces left atrial pressure and relieves congestive heart failure. The procedure may be used as a second choice when balloon atrioseptostomy fails.

Palliative corrective repairs, the Mustard and Senning open-heart procedures, don't correct the anatomic anomaly. However, they permit the right ventricle to continue as the systemic blood circuit, with the left ventricle as the pulmonary blood circuit.

- *Mustard procedure.* Best performed in a patient between age 6 and 36 months, this technique involves suturing a Dacron or pericardial baffle to the excised atrial septum. The baffle redirects pulmonary blood through the tricuspid valve to the right ventricle, and systemic blood through the mitral valve to the left ventricle. The doctor also performs patch closure of the VSD.

- *Senning procedure.* This open-heart surgery uses a coronary sinus flap and an atrial flap instead of a synthetic graft. Atrial tissue serves as the interatrial baffle that directs systemic blood through the mitral valve and pulmonary blood through the tricuspid valve. The tissue grows with the child. However, Blalock-Hanlon septectomy can't be palliatively performed if a Senning procedure's being considered.

- *Anatomic corrective surgery.* The Jatene procedure, a relatively new open-heart surgery, corrects TGV by detaching the coronary arteries from the aorta and transecting the aorta and pulmonary artery above the valves. The doctor then anastomoses the aorta to the pulmonary artery stump and the pulmonary artery to the aortic stump, restoring normal cardiac blood flow. Repair of septal defects, done before the Jatene surgery, permits him to reimplant the coronary arteries onto the new aorta. Candidates for this high-risk surgery must have strong left ventricular function.

Tricuspid atresia

In this defect, an incomplete or absent tricuspid valve prevents blood flow from the right atrium to the right ventricle. Typically, it occurs with an absent or hypoplastic right ventricle, an ASD, or a VSD.

Tricuspid atresia results when the endocardial cushions, a portion of the ventricular septum, and the ventricular muscle fail to merge during the 5th week of gestation. Because the right atrium and ventricle don't communicate, right atrial blood shunts through an atrial septal defect into the left atrium. The unoxygenated blood mixes with oxygenated blood in the left atrium, resulting in cyanosis. If the atrial defect's restricted, right atrial pressure builds, resulting in right heart failure. A concurrent ventricular septal defect causes

Congenital Heart Defects

Tricuspid atresia: A missing valve

An incomplete or absent tricuspid valve prevents blood flow from the right atrium into the right ventricle in this defect. Instead, right atrial blood shunts through an atrial septal defect into the left atrium and then the left ventricle (as shown below). From there, blood travels into the aorta or through a small ventricular defect into the hypoplastic right ventricle, then enters the hypoplastic pulmonary artery.

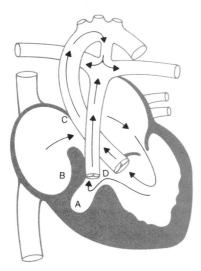

A: Hypoplastic right ventricle
B: Atresia of the tricuspid valve
C: Atrial septal defect
D: Ventricular septal defect

shunting from the left to right ventricle, increasing left ventricular work load. Systemic hypoxemia may occur if pulmonary stenosis decreases pulmonary blood flow. Otherwise, increased pulmonary blood flow may lead to congestive heart failure.

Assessment. Usually, the infant presents with cyanosis and possibly congestive heart failure. As he grows, he may develop pulmonary stenosis or a progressively smaller VSD that may intensify the cyanosis.

Auscultate for a systolic murmur at the second intercostal space along the left border. A single S_1 reflects the absent tricuspid valve; a single S_2, the diminished or absent pulmonic component.

The EKG shows left axis deviation, left and right atrial hypertrophy, and left ventricular hypertrophy. A chest X-ray shows a normal size heart but decreased pulmonary vascular markings. Cardiac catheterization reveals an ASD and increased right atrial pressure. Angiography confirms the diagnosis.

Intervention. Digitalis and diuretics help minimize congestive heart failure, while close monitoring of intake and output helps prevent hemoconcentration. A newborn with a restricted atrial defect who depends on a PDA for pulmonary blood flow may be given prostaglandin E_1 (alprostadil, or Prostin VR) to keep the ductus open until palliative surgery can be performed.

Several palliative surgical procedures can relieve tricuspid atresia. Rashkind balloon atrioseptostomy and Blalock-Hanlon atrial septectomy both augment intraarterial blood flow. The child with congestive heart failure who doesn't respond to medical measures may need pulmonary arterial banding. The doctor may perform a systemic pulmonary artery shunt to increase pulmonary blood flow. If one branch of the pulmonary artery's small, the doctor will choose the Blalock-Taussig shunt. For a child with a small main pulmonary artery, he'll use a central shunt (Waterston or Potts).

Occasionally part of corrective surgery, the Glenn shunt involves anastomosis of the right superior vena cava to the right pulmonary artery. The superior vena cava then receives systemic venous blood from the head and upper torso, shunting it directly to the lungs. As a result, the shunt doesn't increase left ventricular work load. However, the Glenn shunt's not recommended for children younger than age 1 because of its increased mortality risk. This shunt also promotes development of collateral circulation to the inferior vena cava.

The Fontan procedure, corrective surgery for tricuspid atresia, bypasses the right ventricle and directs blood flow to the lungs. Contraindicated for a patient with high pulmonary vascular resistance, the procedure involves two stages: the Glenn shunt followed by a median sternotomy with cardiopulmonary bypass. During the latter, the doctor sews the ASD closed. If the patient has a small right ventricle, the doctor also sews the pulmonic valve closed and places a conduit between the right atrium and left pulmonary artery to carry blood from the inferior vena cava. For a patient without pulmonary stenosis, a conduit between the right atrium and right ventricle presents the better option. Doctors who believe two-stage

Continued on page 154

Congenital Heart Defects

Malposition of the heart

In this defect, the entire heart or one of its segments takes an abnormal position. Assessment of the heart's morphology and its relationship to other organs will reveal the disorder. Major malposition types include dextrocardia, mesocardia, levocardia, and ectopia cordis.

Dextrocardia. In this disorder, the cardiac apex lies on the chest's right side. This defect commonly accompanies noncardiac anomalies, such as situs inversus—transposition of the abdominal viscera.

Mesocardia. In this rare condition, the heart lies in the middle of the chest.

Isolated levocardia. The heart lies in its normal position on the chest's left side, but abdominal visceral organs reverse positions (situs inversus). Cardiac anomalies, such as transposition of the great vessels and double-outlet right ventricle, may also occur.

Ectopia cordis. The heart lies either partially or totally outside the chest in this defect. Ectopia cordis can be thoracic or thoracoabdominal. The latter usually appears with other cardiac anomalies. Treatment of malposition depends on associated anomalies and typically involves corrective surgery.

Cyanotic heart defects—*continued*

corrective surgery isn't necessary recommend directly connecting the right atrium and pulmonary artery, or the right atrium and right ventricle, without the Glenn shunt.

Hypoplastic left ventricle syndrome

Infants with this disorder have an absent or small left ventricle, aortic and/or mitral valve stenosis or atresia, intact ventricular septum, and possibly hypoplasia of the ascending aorta. The syndrome, which results from faulty embryonic heart development, accounts for more deaths in the first 2 weeks of life than any other cardiac defect.

The small left ventricular chamber, combined with aortic or mitral valve obstruction, leads to decreased blood flow to the aorta, resulting in reduced systemic blood flow. Blood backs up in the left atrium, which increases left atrial pressure and engorges the pulmonary vasculature. As left atrial pressure increases, blood shunts from the left to right atrium through a patent foramen ovale, further boosting pulmonary blood flow. A PDA saves the infant's life by supplying systemic blood flow from the right ventricle.

Assessment. Although the neonate may appear normal initially, he rapidly develops tachypnea, dyspnea, a grayish pallor, and cyanosis as the ductus arteriosus begins to close. Eventually, pulmonary engorgement also precipitates respiratory distress, crackles, clammy skin, and hepatomegaly. Most neonates have a nonspecific murmur. Peripheral pulses, normal at first, diminish markedly.

A chest X-ray may show cardiomegaly with increased pulmonary vascular markings. An EKG may be normal or may reveal right ventricular hypertrophy. Echocardiography outlines the small left ventricle.

Detecting complications of corrective surgery

Your patient may develop various complications after corrective congenital heart defect surgery. The chart below shows which signs and symptoms to check for when assessing the patient postoperatively.

Complication	What to check for
Dysrhythmia (heart block)	• abnormal heart rate or rhythm • decreased blood pressure • weak peripheral pulses • pallor or cyanosis
Heart failure	• pulmonary congestion—dyspnea, tachypnea, cough, crackles, abnormal arterial blood gases, increased central venous or pulmonary arterial pressure • venous congestion—distended neck veins, peripheral edema, ascites, enlarged liver, decreased urine output, increased specific gravity, increased blood urea nitrogen (BUN) level • decreased cardiac output
Hematuria	• possible reddish urine • jaundice • increased bilirubin, BUN, and creatinine levels • decreased hemoglobin and hematocrit levels

Continued

Congenital Heart Defects

Pulmonary atresia

This rare defect obstructs right ventricular outflow (the ventricular septum remains intact). A patent ductus arteriosus (PDA) maintains pulmonary blood flow, while an atrial septal defect (ASD) clears right atrial blood. If the patient doesn't have an ASD, the doctor will perform balloon atrial septostomy or septectomy to establish one. Although the neonate may appear normal, he eventually develops cyanosis and tachypnea as the PDA begins to close. The doctor may order prostaglandin E_1 (alprostadil, or Prostin VR) to keep the ductus open until he can surgically construct a systemic pulmonary artery shunt. For a patient with a normal right ventricle, he may perform a valvotomy to open the main pulmonary artery. A patient with a normal pulmonary artery may require a valved prosthetic conduit.

Detecting complications of corrective surgery —continued	
Complication	**What to check for**
Air embolus	• altered level of consciousness • unequal pupils • tachycardia • respiratory distress • seizures • focal neurologic signs
Recurrent laryngeal nerve paralysis	• hoarseness or loss of voice
Phrenic nerve damage	• difficulty in weaning from ventilator • respiratory distress • chronic bronchitis • epigastric discomfort
Chylothorax	• cloudy chest tube drainage
Hemothorax	• tachycardia • decreased blood pressure • dyspnea • decreased breath sounds • clammy skin • weak, thready pulse • bloody chest tube drainage
Paradoxical hypertension	• diastolic blood pressure above 119 mm Hg • headache • flushed skin
Horner's syndrome	• ptosis • miosis • hemifacial loss of sweating • enophthalmos
Mesenteric arteritis	• abdominal pain and distention • diminished bowel sounds • bloody stools
Paraplegia	• decreased sensation and/or mobility in lower torso and legs • loss of bowel/bladder control
Systemic desaturation	• peripheral cyanosis • prolonged capillary refill time • decreased tissue perfusion
Thrombus formation	• shortness of breath • cyanosis • chest pain • loss of consciousness
Vena caval syndrome	• facial edema • pleural effusion • chylothorax • enlarged liver • ascites
Decreased ventricular function	• pulmonary edema • respiratory distress • shortness of breath

Intervention. Most neonates receive only symptomatic therapy—prostaglandin E_1—to keep the ductus arteriosus patent and to maintain systemic blood flow. However, several experimental surgical procedures aim to increase systemic blood flow while decreasing blood flow to the left atrium. Initially, surgery involves anastomosis of the diminutive ascending aorta to the proximal main pulmonary artery, establishing a systemic pulmonary shunt. When the child begins to outgrow this shunt, the doctor will perform a second

Continued on page 156

Congenital Heart Defects

Cyanotic heart defects—*continued*

procedure called a modified Fontan. This consists of removing the systemic pulmonary shunt and creating an intraatrial baffle, which directs left atrial blood flow through the tricuspid valve via an ASD. The doctor then directly anastomoses the right atrium to the pulmonary artery. This corrective surgery establishes independent pulmonary and systemic blood circuits.

Self Test

1. When caring for a child with a cyanotic congenital heart defect, take special precautions with I.V. lines to prevent air embolus caused by:
a. right-to-left shunting of oxygenated blood   **b.** left-to-right shunting of oxygenated blood   **c.** right-to-left shunting of unoxygenated blood   **d.** left-to-right shunting of unoxygenated blood

2. If you auscultate a "machinery" murmur during systole and diastole, suspect:
a. coarctation of the aorta   **b.** ventricular septal defect   **c.** tetralogy of Fallot   **d.** patent ductus arteriosus

3. Tet spells may occur after activities that:
a. increase systemic resistance   **b.** decrease systemic resistance   **c.** increase oxygen demand   **d.** decrease oxygen demand

4. Prostaglandin E_1 (alprostadil, or Prostin VR) can help treat patent ductus arteriosus by:
a. increasing systemic blood flow   **b.** decreasing systemic blood flow   **c.** closing the ductus   **d.** dilating the ductus

Answers (page number shows where answer appears in text)

1. **c** (page 142)   2. **d** (page 146)   3. **c** (page 149)   4. **d** (page 145—*A role for drugs*)

Selected References

Books

Barry, Anna. *Aortic and Tricuspid Valvular Disease.* East Norwalk, Conn.: Appleton-Century-Crofts, 1980.

Bates, Barbara. *A Guide to Physical Examination,* 3rd ed. Philadelphia: J.B. Lippincott Co., 1983.

Braunwald, Eugene, ed. *Heart Disease: A Textbook of Cardiovascular Medicine,* 2 vols., 2nd ed. Philadelphia: W.B. Saunders Co., 1984.

Cardiac Crises. Nursing Now Series. Springhouse, Pa.: Springhouse Corp., 1984.

Carpenito, Lynda J. *Nursing Diagnosis: Application to Clinical Practice.* Philadelphia: J.B. Lippincott Co., 1983.

Chung, Edward K. *Quick Reference to Cardiovascular Diseases,* 2nd ed. Philadelphia: J.B. Lippincott Co., 1982.

Conover, Mary B. *Understanding Electrocardiography: Arrhythmias and the 12-Lead ECG,* 4th ed. St. Louis: C.V. Mosby Co., 1984.

Dalen, James E., and Alpert, Joseph E. *Valvular Heart Disease.* Boston: Little, Brown & Co., 1981.

Fowler, Noble O. *Cardiac Diagnosis and Treatment,* 3rd ed. Philadelphia: J.B. Lippincott Co., 1980.

Guido, Virginia. *Septal Defects: Atrial and Ventricular.* East Norwalk, Conn.: Appleton-Century-Crofts, 1982.

Guzzetta, Cathie E., and Dossey, Barbara M. *Cardiovascular Disease Nursing: Bodymind Tapestry.* St. Louis: C.V. Mosby Co., 1984.

Hillis, L. David, and Firth, Brian G. *Manual of Clinical Problems in Cardiology,* 2nd ed. Boston: Little, Brown & Co., 1984.

Horwitz, Lawrence D., and Graves, Bertron M. *Signs and Symptoms in Cardiology.* Philadelphia: J.B. Lippincott Co., 1985.

Hurst, J. Willis, ed. *The Heart, Arteries and Veins.* New York: McGraw-Hill Book Co., 1982.

Johanson, Brenda C., et al. *Standards for Critical Care.* St. Louis: C.V. Mosby Co., 1981.

Marriot, Henry J., and Conover, Mary H. *Advanced Concepts in Arrhythmias.* St. Louis: C.V. Mosby Co., 1983.

Michaelson, Cydney R., ed. *Congestive Heart Failure.* St. Louis: C.V. Mosby Co., 1983.

Moller, James H., and Neal, William A. *Heart Disease in Infancy.* East Norwalk, Conn.: Appleton-Century-Crofts, 1981.

Opie, Lionel H., ed. et al. *Drugs for the Heart: American Edition.* New York: Grune and Stratton, 1984.

Sadler, D., ed. *Nursing for Cardiovascular Health.* East Norwalk, Conn.: Appleton-Century-Crofts, 1983.

Stark, J., and DeLeval, M., eds. *Surgery for Congenital Heart Defects in Infants.* New York: Grune and Stratton, 1983.

Sweetwood, Hannelore. *Clinical Electrocardiography for Nurses.* Rockville, Md.: Aspen Systems Corp., 1983.

Thompson, June M., and Bowers, Arden C. *Clinical Manual of Health Assessment.* St. Louis: C.V. Mosby Co., 1980.

Underhill, Sandra L., and Woods, Susan L. *Cardiac Nursing.* Philadelphia: J.B. Lippincott Co., 1982.

Periodicals

Kienzle, M.G., et al. "Antiarrhythmic Drug Therapy for Sustained Ventricular Tachycardia," *Heart and Lung* 13(6):614-22, November 1984.

Ludmer, P.L., and Goldschlager, N. "Cardiac Pacing in the 1980's," *New England Journal of Medicine* 311(26):1671-80, December 1984.

Parker, M.M., and Lemberg, L. "Pacemaker Update 1984. Part I, Introduction to Electrocardiographic Analysis of Pacing Function and Site," *Heart and Lung* 13(3):315-18, May 1984.

Willoughby, M.L., and Dunlap, D.B. "The Treatment of Atrial Fibrillation and Flutter: A Review," *Heart and Lung* 13(5):578-84, September 1984.

Index

i refers to an illustration; t to a table

Index

i refers to an illustration; t to a table

Index

i refers to an illustration; t to a table